Advances in Diagnosis and Therapy of Colorectal Carcinoma

Edited by Jindong Chen

Published in London, United Kingdom

Advances in Diagnosis and Therapy of Colorectal Carcinoma
http://dx.doi.org/10.5772/intechopen.1001498
Edited by Jindong Chen

Contributors
Ali Kaan Güren, Amido Rey, Ana Druzijanic, Ardaman Shergill, Gede Eka Rusdi Antara, Gui-Qin Wang, Guodong Tie, Imelda Rey, Ivana Vucenik, Jing Zhang, Louis Messina, Marcus Marable, Min-Yi Wu, Muriel Battaglia, Nikica Druzijanic, Osman Köstek, Qi Xie, Rustam Effendi-YS, Susan L. Feldt, Veysel Cem Ozcan, Xi-Yan Shao, Yi-Ming Yang

First published in London, United Kingdom, 2024 by IntechOpen
IntechOpen is the global imprint of INTECHOPEN LIMITED, registered in England and Wales, registration number: 11086078, 167-169 Great Portland Street, London, W1W 5PF, United Kingdom

British Library Cataloguing-in-Publication Data
A catalogue record for this book is available from the British Library

Additional hard and PDF copies can be obtained from orders@intechopen.com

Advances in Diagnosis and Therapy of Colorectal Carcinoma
Edited by Jindong Chen
p. cm.
Print ISBN 978-0-85466-614-0
Online ISBN 978-0-85466-613-3
eBook (PDF) ISBN 978-0-85466-615-7

Meet the editor

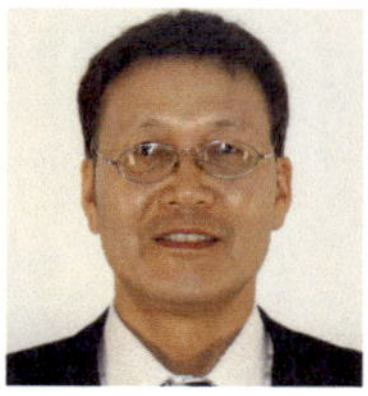

Jindong Chen obtained his Ph.D. from the Karolinska Institute, Sweden. He is an active member of the American Association for Cancer Research (AACR) and the chief technology officer at Exploring Health, LLC. He is a former associate professor and kidney laboratory co-director at the University of Rochester Medical Center, USA. When serving as a research scientist at Van Andel Research Institute, USA, and a senior scientist at the National Cancer Center Singapore and Duke-NUS University Medical School, USA, Dr. Chen position-cloned two cancer-related genes, NORE1 and LSAMP, and participated in the identification of HRPT2 and FLCN. He subsequently developed several FLCN and HRPT2 knockout mouse models. For those achievements, he was awarded at the 94th and 100th AACR annual meetings. To date, he has published more than 120 papers and 4 academic monographs/books. Currently, Dr. Chen is working on the development of anti-metastasis drugs and has been granted more than 20 patents.

Contents

Preface

Colorectal cancer is the third most common cancer globally, accounting for approximately 10% of all cancer cases, and it ranks as the second leading cause of cancer-related deaths worldwide. In 2020, more than 1.9 million new cases of colorectal cancer and more than 930,000 deaths due to colorectal cancer were estimated to have occurred worldwide. By 2040, the burden of colorectal cancer will increase to 3.2 million new cases per year (an increase of 63%) and 1.6 million deaths per year (an increase of 73%). Colorectal cancer is often diagnosed at advanced stages when treatment options are limited. With the development and improvement of new techniques, updated knowledge and information are essential for management of colorectal cancer.

In the past decade, the use of improved diagnostic methods such as endoscopy, abdominal ultrasound, computed tomography (CT), magnetic resonance imaging (MRI), positron emission tomography (PET), and liquid biopsy (tumor cell or nucleic acid-based molecular detection method) has significantly increased the detection rate of colorectal cancer. Additionally, surgical treatment remains the first-line treatment to provide a cure, and advances in surgery, including robotic surgical systems, have partly solved several constraints of laparoscopic surgery. These new techniques offer technical advantages in colorectal cancer surgery, which has improved the outcome of surgical treatment, and their application will further expand in the future. For advanced or metastatic colorectal cancer, the progress in targeted therapy, immunotherapy, cellular directed therapy, and combination therapy has been improving patient survival outcomes. For these reasons, the mortality of colorectal cancer in the future is expected to decrease.

With international experts sharing their valuable experience, knowledge, and reviews on these various aspects in the management of colorectal cancer, this book offers all physicians treating colorectal cancer, as well as researchers, updated information on the epidemiology, diagnosis, and recent advances in treatment and management of colorectal cancer. It is also a valuable resource for other specialists, researchers, and colorectal cancer patients.

I would like to give my sincere and hearty thanks to all the chapter authors for their excellent contributions. I would also like to thank the staff at IntechOpen, especially Publishing Process Manager Ms. Valentina Jolić. Without these individuals, this book would not have been possible.

Jindong Chen
Chief Technology Officer,
Exploring Health, LLC,
Guangzhou, China

Section 1

Diangnosis of Colorectal Cancer

Chapter 1

Challenges of Colorectal Screening in Developing Countries

Gede Eka Rusdi Antara

Abstract

Colorectal cancer (CRC) is the third most common cancer worldwide in 2020. Screening is especially suitable for colorectal cancer (CRC), given its prevalence and the belief that it represents a progressive adenoma-carcinoma chain. In developing nations, CRC screening is occasionally opportunistic; it is sometimes detected concurrently with other symptoms. There are several simple screening methods available such as digital rectal examination and fecal occult blood test (FOBT). Furthermore, the more advance screening method endoscopic, stoll-based, or radiological, blood-based screening also available. But in the developing countries, that options are limited due to lack of data, knowledge, awareness, human resources, infrastructure, screening guidelines, and cost issue. To overcome that challenge, technological development, policy updates, and the right screening choice can be effective in that setting.

Keywords: colorectal cancer, challenge, developing country, screening, cancer, CRC

1. Introduction

Following lung and breast cancer in terms of frequency of diagnosis, colorectal cancer (CRC) is the third most common cancer worldwide in 2020. In 2020, CRC came in third place for men and second place for women. A total of 1.931.590 new cases, or 10.01% of the total, are diagnosed annually [1]. In Asia, colorectal cancer accounted for 1,009,400 (17.6%) incidents and 506,449 (8.7%) deaths of all sexes and ages. CRC is becoming an increasing health concern, particularly in developing nations. An environmental factor significantly affects the pathogenesis of colorectal cancer (CRC), as evidenced by the greater than 10-fold variation in global CRC incidence and the rapid increase in CRC risk among the same generation of immigrants from low-risk to high-risk regions [2].

Colorectal cancer (CRC) is an intestinal or rectal disorder. It results from an abnormal proliferation of glandular epithelial cells in the colon. Sporadic, hereditary, and colitis-related are the three primary classifications of CRC [3]. Cases of CRC are on the rise worldwide. Genetic and environmental factors influence the likelihood of developing CRC. Furthermore, patients who have ulcerative colitis and Crohn's disease have an elevated risk of developing colorectal cancer (CRC) as they age [4]. Several studies identify diet and lifestyle, family history, and chronic inflammation as risk factors for CRC [4]. CRC cases have increased in economically developed nations due to the adoption of Western lifestyles and dietary habits, which are marked by excessive consumption of meat, fat, and total calories. Population growth and an extended life expectancy have also contributed to this trend [3, 5].

Screening is especially suitable for colorectal cancer (CRC), given its prevalence and the belief that it represents a progressive adenoma-carcinoma chain. While the precise duration from initial adenoma to established colorectal cancer (CRC) remains unknown, available evidence indicates that it should not fall below 10 years. This provides ample time for early detection via screening and subsequent treatment. Moreover, colorectal adenomas can be removed to prevent colorectal cancer (CRC), and early detection of CRC reduces the patient's mortality risk [6]. In patients devoid of symptoms and at no risk, fecal tests (FOBT) and fecal immunochemical tests (FIT) are the most frequently advised and implemented screening methods for colorectal cancer (CRC). These tests are specifically designed to identify minute quantities of blood in the stool. Screening programs in high-income countries commonly invite all individuals aged 50 and above to participate by submitting a stool sample. This strategy is not yet fully implemented in developing nations due to inadequate infrastructure and resources [7].

In developing nations, CRC screening is occasionally opportunistic; it is sometimes detected concurrently with other symptoms. Frequently, CRC cases are identified after the onset of symptoms. Screening is crucial for preventing CRC-related mortality and morbidity. Conquering the high mortality rate associated with colorectal cancer (CRC) and the dearth of screening services in developing nations represents a formidable obstacle [8]. Colorectal cancer is a malignant disease that requires the establishment and implementation of screening interventions if it is not detected early. Hence, this literature review aims to examine the obstacles associated with colorectal cancer screening in developing nations.

2. CRC epidemiology in developing countries

Based on 2018 GLOBOCAN data, colon cancer is the malignancy with the fourth highest incidence in the world, while rectal cancer is the eighth-highest malignancy in the world. When combined, the incidence of colorectal cancer (CRC) is the third highest in the world, with an estimated 11% of all diagnosed cancers. In 2018, there were more than 1 million new cases of colon cancer and more than 700 thousand new cases of rectal cancer, with an estimated more than 1.8 million new cases of CRC diagnosed [9].

Based on demographics, the incidence of CRC in men is higher than in women, 3–4 times, and is more common in developed countries than in developing countries. The age-standardized incidence rate per 100,000 CRC cases for both sexes is 19.7, lower than the rate of 23.6 for men and higher than 16.3 for women. The age-standardized incidence for men in countries with a high human development index (HDI) is 30.1 per 100,000, while in low-HDI countries it is only 8.4 per 100,000 [9].

Several recent studies show that CRC incidence and mortality increases in countries with medium-high HDI. This is associated with sedentary lifestyle habits, obesity, red meat consumption, smoking habits, and alcohol consumption. Furthermore, the CRC incidence rate in these countries is also increasing along with increasing life expectancy [10]. In general, the incidence of CRC in developing countries or low-HDI nations also varies. Age-standardized rate (ASR) incidence and mortality figures for several regions in the world can be seen in the **Table 1**.

Region/Category	ASR Incidence	ASR Mortality
Medium-HDI countries	11.3	6.7
Low-HDI countries	4.9	3.9
Micronesia	20.4	8.3
Eastern Asia	18.4	8.4
Caribbean	16.4	9.1
Polynesia	15.0	6.6
South-Eastern Asia	12.5	7.9
Southern Africa	10.9	7.4
Melanesia	8.8	6.2
Northern Africa	7.6	5.0
Eastern Africa	6.5	5.0
South-Central Asia	6.1	4.4
Sub-Saharan Africa	5.8	4.5
Middle Africa	4.8	3.9
Western Africa	4.1	3.3

**ASR per 100.000 cases [11].*

Table 1.
Age-standardized rate for incidence and mortality of CRC in developing countries [11].

Although in general the incidence of CRC is lower in developing countries, recent trends show that the incidence of CRC in several developing countries has increased. The incidence rate in several former Eastern European Communist Bloc countries which are currently undergoing major economic transitions has equaled or exceeded the incidence in several developed countries of the former Western Bloc. The same thing is also observed in several countries in the East Asia region such as Taiwan, Hong Kong, Singapore, China, and Thailand which are showing a drastic increase in the incidence of CRC, so that it is almost close to the incidence rate in European countries [12–15].

An increase in the incidence of CRC has also been found in several West Asian countries which historically have had low incidence rates. Research in Iran shows a drastic increase in incidents in the last 3 decades. Similar things were also found in several other countries in the region such as Jordan, Saudi Arabia, Egypt, and Yemen. An increase in incidents was also found in India, although at a less significant rate compared to several developing countries in the East Asian region [12, 16].

The increase in CRC incidence in several developing countries is not due to an increase in screening rates, because existing screening programs are generally still limited or have only just been implemented in these developing countries. The incidence of CRC was also found to be more common in the young population who were not the target of the screening program. This phenomenon appears to be found in several countries that are experiencing an epidemiological transition, such as Iran, where almost 20% of CRC cases are less than 40 years old [12, 16, 17].

3. Screening of CRC in developing countries

3.1 Indications for colorectal screening

The American Cancer Society (ACS) has published recommendations for routine screening of at-risk individuals starting at age 45 years. Individuals who are considered to have an average risk of colorectal cancer are patients who have no previous history of colorectal cancer or certain types of polyps, no family history of colorectal cancer, no history of inflammatory bowel disease (ulcerative colitis or Crohn's disease), no confirmed history of the colorectal cancer syndrome, and no history of exposure to radiation to the abdomen or pelvic region for cancer treatment. Individuals who have a healthy body condition and have a life expectancy of more than 10 years are encouraged to undergo colorectal cancer screening until the age of 75 years. For individuals aged 76 to 85, the decision to undergo screening is adjusted to general health conditions, life expectancy, patient preferences, and prior screening history. Meanwhile, patients over 85 years of age should no longer receive colorectal cancer screening [18]. In Indonesia, indications for early examination for colorectal cancer are categorized into moderate-risk and high-risk individuals. The indications of screening for individuals classified as moderate risk are as follows [19].

1. Individuals aged 50 years or older.
2. Individuals who do not have a history of colorectal cancer or inflammatory bowel disease (IBD).
3. Individuals who do not have a family history of colorectal cancer
4. Individuals diagnosed with adenoma or colorectal cancer after the age of 60 years

Meanwhile, indications for early detection of colorectal cancer with increased or high risk are as follows [19].

1. Individuals with a history of curative resection of colorectal cancer
2. Individuals with a history of adenomatous polyps
3. Individuals with a long history of inflammatory bowel disease
4. Individuals with a first-degree family history of colorectal cancer or colorectal adenoma. However, these recommendations differ based on the age of the family at diagnosis.
5. Individuals with a diagnosis or suspicion of having Hereditary Non-Polyposis Colorectal Cancer (HNPCC) syndrome or Lynch syndrome or Familial Adenomatous Polyposis (FAP).

Each cancer risk level has a recommended time to start screening and recommendations for examinations to be carried out. Patients with a history of polyps will have their number and grading assessed. In detail, indications, screening start time, and screening recommendations are contained in the following **Table 2** [19].

No.	Risk Categories	Time	Recommendations
1.	Increased risk – Patients with a history of polyps on previous colonoscopy		
	Patients with small hyperplastic polyps	—	Colonoscopy or other screening methods at recommended intervals in moderate-risk individuals
	Patients with 1 or 2 tubular adenomas classified as low-grade dysplasia	5–10 years after initial polypectomy	Colonoscopy
	Patients with 3–10 adenomas or 1 adenoma measuring >1 cm or all with villous/high-grade dysplasia	3 years after initial polypectomy	Colonoscopy every 5 years
	Patients who had >10 adenomas at one examination	<3 years after initial polypectomy	Colonoscopy
	Patients who had sessile adenomas removed at one time	22–6 months to ensure complete removal	Colonoscopy. Complete or incomplete removal is subject to endoscopic and pathological assessment.
2.	Increased risk – Patients with colorectal cancer		
	Colon and rectal cancer patients who should undergo high-quality perioperative clearance	3–6 months after cancer resection if unresectable metastases are not found	Colonoscopy
	Patients undergoing curative resection for colon and rectal cancer	1-year post-resection	Colonoscopy
3.	Increased risk – Patients with family history		
	First-degree relatives before the age of 60 years have a history of colorectal cancer or adenomatous polyps or ≥ 2 first-degree relatives at any age.	Age 40 years or 10 years before the youngest case in the family	Colonoscopy every 5 years
	A history of colorectal cancer or adenomatous polyps in a first-degree relative >60 years or 2 second-degree family members with colorectal cancer	At the age of 40 years	Screening methods and intervals are adjusted to moderate risk recommendations.
4	High risk		
	Individuals diagnosed with FAP without evidence of genetic testing	Age 10–12 years	Sigmoidoscopy every 1 year to assess abnormal genetic expression. If the genetic test is positive, then consider a colectomy.
	Patients with a genetic or clinical diagnosis suggestive of HNPCC or patients at increased risk of HNPCC	Age 20–25 years or 10 years before the youngest case in the family was discovered	Colonoscopy every 1–2 years. At HNPCC, genetic testing is considered.
	Patients with IBD, Crohn's disease, or chronic ulcerative colitis	8 years after pancolitis or 12–15 years after onset of left-sided colitis	Colonoscopy every 1–2 years and biopsy to assess for dysplasia

Table 2.
Indications of screening based on risk categories and recommendations of examination [19].

3.2 Early detection in individuals with suspected colorectal cancer

Simple screening methods that are often used to check for colorectal cancer are digital rectal examination and fecal occult blood test (FOBT).

3.2.1 Digital rectal examination

Based on the guidelines published by the Indonesian Ministry of Health, a digital rectal examination can be performed once on individuals over 50 years. If clinical symptoms appear, a re-examination can be carried out [19]. The purpose of a digital rectal examination is to evaluate the presence of abnormalities in the perianal, distal rectum, anal canal, and rectovaginal septum in women. Apart from that, this examination also aims to determine the integrity of the anal sphincter and determine the size and degree of tumor fixation in the middle and distal 1/3 of the rectum. Specifically for colorectal cancer, the points assessed are the condition of the tumor, tumor mobility, extension, and tumor size. What is evaluated from the condition of the tumor are the extension of the lesion on the rectal wall and the location of the lowest part of the uterine cervix, the anorectal ring, and the top of the prostate. Tumor mobility is assessed to determine the surgical therapy to be performed. Meanwhile, tumor extension is observed by evaluating the upper, lower, and circular borders [19, 20].

The health care provider performs a rectal exam by first asking about the symptoms of the rectum, such as bleeding, pain, or a palpable mass. The examiner then assesses the condition of the perianal with a radius of 5 cm from the anal verge, followed by 360° palpation of the anal canal and distal rectum. This examination is relatively fast and generally does not exceed 1 minute. Apart from the fast examination time, this examination is also cost-effective as a colorectal cancer screening [20, 21].

The digital rectal examination is more useful for determining distal rectal tumors [19]. Research conducted by Tanaka et al. also found that digital rectal examination was more accurate in determining lower rectal lesions than middle rectal lesions. His research found that digital rectal examination tends to give a lower estimated height than endoscopy above 7 cm from the anal verge. A rectal digital examination can provide information regarding the depth of invasion and circumferential location of colorectal cancer [22]. However, this digital rectal examination depends on the expertise and experience of the examining doctor. It is also limited to the reach of the examining finger. The other study stated that digital rectal examination is not suitable for tumors that are >10 cm from the edge of the anal. Therefore, a digital rectal examination is more accurate in determining locally advanced stages than early tumor stages [19, 22].

3.2.2 Fecal occult blood tests (FOBTs)

The other early detection is fecal occult blood tests (FOBTs). This examination is useful for detecting early-stage colorectal cancer. FOBT is an examination used to detect the presence of blood in feces that cannot be seen with a microscope. Currently, there are three types of FOBT based on measurement techniques: chemical tests, immunochromatography tests, and DNA tests [23–25].

The gFOBTs examination is a qualitative examination that utilizes the activity of the haem pseudo-peroxidase enzyme from hemoglobin molecules found in feces. The discovery of blood components in feces is caused when haem originating from the blood mediates the oxidation of guaiac acid by hydrogen peroxide to become guaiac blue. However, examination with gFOBTs has a high risk of false positive results [23, 26]. Before undergoing gFOBTs examination, patients are asked to avoid consuming red meat 2–7 days before the test to avoid false positive results. In addition, green vegetables that have chlorophyll-mediated pseudo-peroxidase activity or other foods high in peroxidase are also avoided. These requirements are considered difficult for some patients [25]. Apart from that, the specificity of gFOBTs is also low, namely almost 50%, because positive gFOBT results are not caused by colorectal cancer but by other causes. Therefore, further examination is needed. If an individual has abnormalities in the digital rectum and FOBT, the individual will be referred for further examination [19].

An alternative to gFOBTs testing is 3,3′,5,5′-tetramethylbenzidine (TMB) testing. The TBM examination is a one-stage examination using an examination paper. Paper soaked with TMB indicator is placed in the toilet bowl immediately after defecation. Another step is to stick the patient's finger in the circular area on the front side, then wipe the buttocks to collect a stool specimen in the circular area on the backside. Next, the 3,3′,5,5′-tetramethylbenzidine regimen and the hydrogen peroxide with ethanol regimen will be dripped [27]. In this examination, haem originating from free hemoglobin, myoglobin, or lysed erythrocytes will catalyze the oxidation reaction and trigger a change in action to green or blue within 2 minutes. Compared to gFOBTs, this examination is more comfortable for patients. However, this test only detects blood in the external layer of the feces. Similar to gFOBTs, patients are also asked to avoid consuming red meat, green vegetables, medicines, and citrus fruit 3 days before the examination. Apart from that, the reading of the test results is not objective but is based on the observation. As a result, wrong interpretations can occur, especially if the patient sees the test results from a considerable distance (**Figure 1** and 2) [25, 27].

3.3 Advanced screening in individuals with suspected colorectal cancer

In the United States, several professional communities recommend CRC screening for asymptomatic individuals with an average risk between the ages of 50 and 75 years old [28]. Although the latest guidelines from the American Cancer Society suggest initiating CRC screening at the age of 45 [29]. Commonly used methods include endoscopic methods (colonoscopy and sigmoidoscopy), radiologic methods

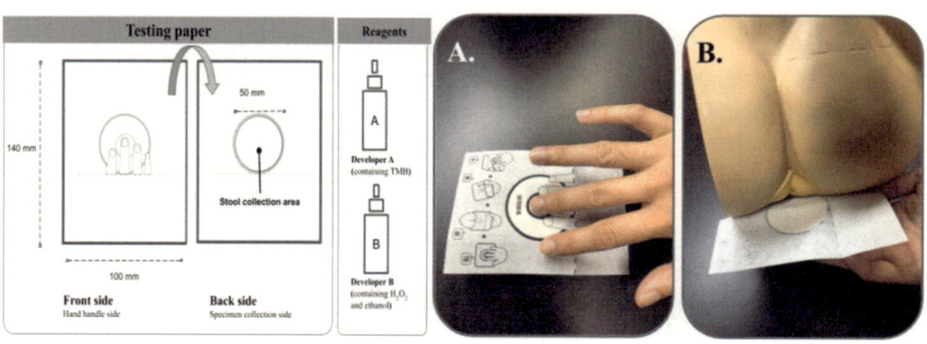

Figure 1.
Design of the toilet paper by TMB test. (A) the front side of the paper. (B) the backside of the paper to collect the stool [27].

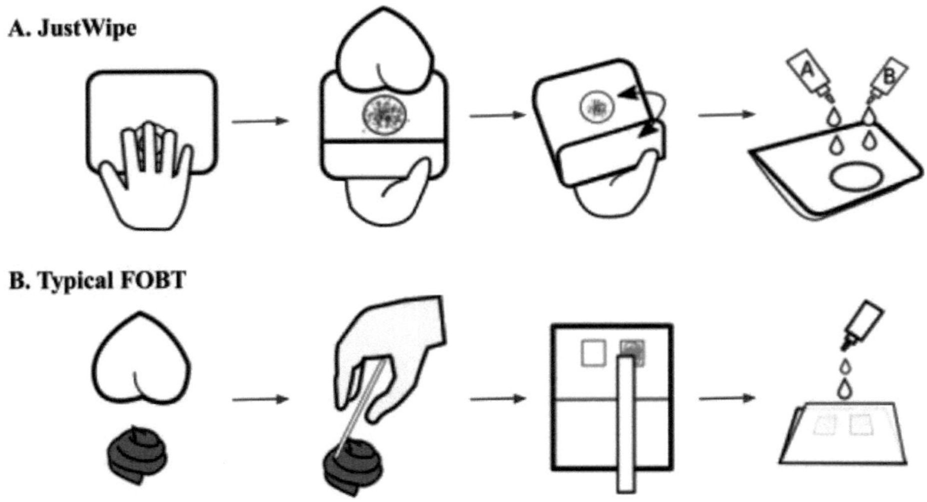

Figure 2.
The comparison between the TMB test and gFOBTs [27].

(computed tomography (CT) colonography), stool-based testing (fecal immunochemical test (FIT) and FIT-DNA), and blood-based screening tests (**Figure 3**) [30].

3.3.1 Endoscopic methods

Endoscopic methods are considered the most sensitive for CRC screening as they allow direct mucosal inspection throughout the large intestine. A thin, flexible, lighted tube is inserted through the anus and used to directly inspect the lining of the rectum and the entire colon. In a population-based case-control study in Germany, a history of colonoscopy resulted in a 77% decreased risk of CRC. In a large population-based case-control study in Canada, colonoscopy reduced mortality rates by 67% [30]. In a large cohort study in the United States with a follow-up period of more than 22 years, negative colonoscopy results were associated with an overall 56% reduction in CRC risk and a 27% reduction in proximal CRC risk [31]. The difference between the reduction in proximal and distal CRC risks is likely related to several factors, including incomplete colonoscopy evaluation, difficult visualization in the proximal colon, poor bowel preparation, and operator skill. Several ongoing large randomized trials are expected to yield important information in the coming years regarding the efficacy of colonoscopy in reducing CRC incidence and mortality. Drawbacks of colonoscopy include discomfort during bowel preparation before the procedure, sedation risks (such as cardiovascular events), and procedure-related complications (such as colon perforation and bleeding). In meta-analyses, there were reported risks of perforation (0.5 per 1000), post-colonoscopy bleeding (2.6 per 1000), and mortality (2.9 per 100,000). Because the procedure usually requires sedation, you must be accompanied home after the procedure, and you should not return to work or other activities on the same day. The complication rates were found to be lower for screening procedures compared to diagnostic examinations [30, 32].

Another advanced screening method is flexible sigmoidoscopy, which examines the lower part of the colon. Several studies indicate a decrease in CRC incidence among individuals undergoing sigmoidoscopy followed by colonoscopy compared to those

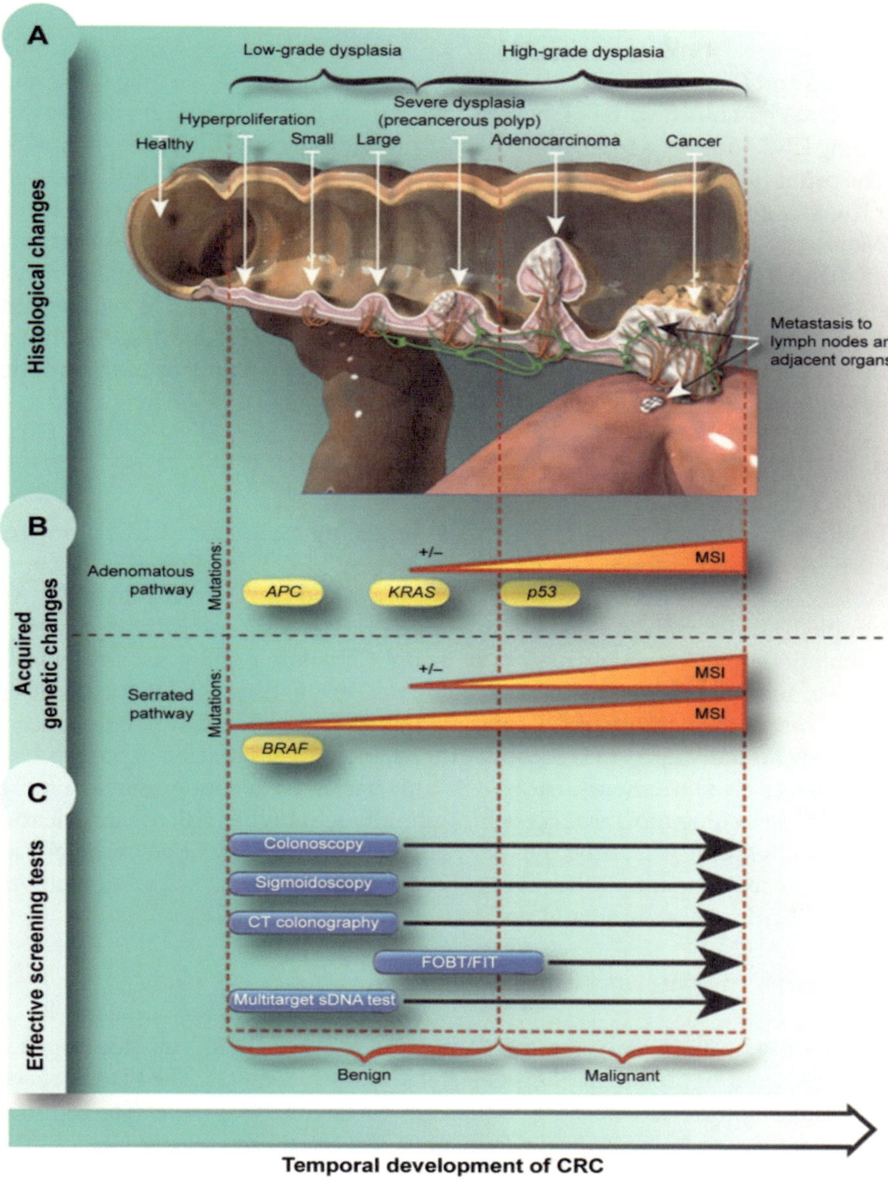

Figure 3.
CRC development and screening methods [44]. CRC, colorectal cancer; CIMP, CpG island methylator phenotype; CT, computed tomography; FOBT, fecal occult blood test; FIT, fecal immunochemical test; MSI, microsatellite instability; sDNA, stool DNA.

without screening. A major disadvantage of sigmoidoscopy is that it cannot detect polyps or cancers that are located only on the right side (for example, in the cecum or ascending colon to the hepatic flexure) or in the transverse colon, which are more common in older women [33]. In a large multicenter randomized trial in the UK with a 17-year follow-up, there was a 26% reduction in CRC incidence and a 30% decrease in CRC-related mortality [34]. Sigmoidoscopy remains a suitable choice for CRC screening when colonoscopy availability is limited. The United States Preventive Services Task Force (USPSTF) recommends screening with flexible sigmoidoscopy every 5 years [35].

3.3.2 Stool-based testing

The Food and Drug Administration (FDA) recommends CRC screening using multi-target Fit-DNA combined with FIT. Fit-DNA testing has proven to have higher sensitivity in detecting CRC compared to FIT (92.3 vs. 73.8%) but lower specificity (86.6 vs. 94.9%) [36]. The primary drawback of FIT-DNA lies in its lower specificity than FIT, leading to a higher likelihood of false-positive results, necessitating further examination via colonoscopy. Moreover, data regarding the mortality benefits of FIT-DNA as a CRC screening test remain limited. Although the Centers for Medicare & Medicaid Services approve and recommend FIT-DNA at three-year intervals in the United States, the optimal frequency for using FIT-DNA for CRC screening has not been definitively established. Additionally, the cost of FIT-DNA is significantly higher than FIT, which might pose a barrier to adopting this screening method in developing countries [30].

3.3.3 Radiologic method

CT Colonography is a radiologically-based screening method for CRC. Compared to barium enemas, CT colonography is more sensitive [37]. CT colonography can detect adenomas ≥1 cm with a sensitivity of 67–94% and specificity of 86–98% [38, 39]. European studies indicate that CT colonography has a high sensitivity comparable to colonoscopy for polyps larger than 5 mm. CT colonography also presents the advantage of minimal risk of perforation compared to colonoscopy [40]. However, for smaller polyps, the sensitivity of CT colonography is lower than that of colonoscopy. There are several drawbacks to CT colonography, including radiation exposure and bowel preparation requirements. Despite its drawbacks, CT colonography is a recommended CRC screening tool, especially for individuals at higher risk of complications related to colonoscopy. Presently, the U.S. Multi-Society Task Force recommends a CT colonography screening interval of every 5 years, and individuals with colon polyps ≥6 mm on CT colonography should undergo colonoscopy [28, 30].

3.3.4 Blood-based screening tests (liquid biopsy)

Liquid biopsy involves analyzing circulating tumor cells (CTCs), cell-free tumor DNA (ctDNA), and/or protein markers detectable in the blood [41]. The FDA approved the first serum test for CRC screening, which is methylated DNA septin9. The septin9 test has a sensitivity of 48.2% and specificity of 91.5%. Sensitivity for CRC stages I-IV is 35.0, 63.0, 46.0, and 77.4%, respectively, but sensitivity for advanced adenomas is only 11.2% [42]. The Septin9 test has the advantage of being more comfortable for patients, thereby increasing their willingness to undergo screening. However, the primary drawback of the Septin9 test is its low sensitivity in detecting CRC and its relatively poor performance in detecting advanced adenomas [43]. A meta-analysis involving 14 studies indicated that the sensitivity of Septin9 in diagnosing CRC is only 67, with 89% specificity in distinguishing CRC patients from cancer-free individuals (**Table 3**) [45].

3.4 Screening facilities in developing countries

In developing countries, there is a lack of standard screening and diagnostic facilities, leading to frequent delays in cancer diagnosis. Screening facilities within health care services provided at public facilities were identified as major barriers to screening

Test	Premise	Sensitivity for CRC	Screening interval	Advantages	Limitations
Colonoscopy	Endoscopic examination of the entire colon	>95%	Every 10 years	High sensitivity, allows visualization of full colon, detection of distal and proximal lesions, can remove lesions at time of detection	Invasive, unpleasant bowel preparation, requires special facilities and sedation, cost, accessibility, need for anesthesia, low patient compliance, risk of bowel perforation or bleeding
Sigmoidoscopy	Endoscopic examination of the distal colon	>95% (distal colon only)	Every 5 years in combination with FOBT	High sensitivity (distal colon only), full sedation not required, can remove lesions at time of detection	Semi-invasive, unpleasant bowel preparation, requires special facilities and sedation, cost, accessibility, only screens distal colon, safety concerns, patient discomfort
CT colonography	Radiologic visualization of the colon, aka virtual colonoscopy	>90%	Every 5 years	High sensitivity, allows visualization of full colon, no sedation needed, detection of distal and proximal lesions	Semi-invasive, unpleasant bowel preparation, requires special facilities, cannot remove lesions at time of detection, radiological safety concerns
FOBT	Enzymatic detection of hemoglobin in the stool	33–75%	Annually	Accessibility, noninvasive, low cost, detection of distal and proximal CRC	Poor detection of precancerous lesions, cannot remove lesions at time of detection, detects ingested hemoglobin

Test	Premise	Sensitivity for CRC	Screening interval	Advantages	Limitations
FIT	Immunochemical detection of hemoglobin in the stool	60–85%	Annually	Accessibility, noninvasive, low cost, detection of distal and proximal CRC	Poor detection of precancerous lesions, cannot remove lesions at time of detection
mt-sDNA test	Molecular detection of DNA aberrations and hemoglobin	92%	Every 3 years	High sensitivity, accessibility, noninvasive, detection of proximal and distal lesions	Better detection of cancer than precancerous lesions, cannot remove lesions at time of detection

Table 3.
Advanced screening test for CRC [44].

in developing countries [46]. In developed countries, colonoscopy enjoys better service accessibility and quality, largely owing to adequate resources and stringent quality monitoring. However, in developing countries, the capacity for colonoscopy screening for CRC remains severely limited, as observed in Brazil, Indonesia, and several African nations. Insufficient capacity to conduct colonoscopies, including infrastructure, utilization, and quality, could adversely affect clinical practice and restrict the effectiveness of endoscopic screening in reducing the burden of Colorectal Cancer [47–49]. Currently, the standard imaging technique for staging CRC is a Computed Tomography scan. In the public sector of Tanzania, there are 5.7 radiography units per million population. This figure is significantly lower than the 20 units per million population recommended by the WHO. In developing countries, laboratories for CRC sample testing require more standard equipment and trained clinical pathologists. There is a shortage of gastroenterologists and colonoscopy units in LMICs, especially in rural areas. Consequently, when specimens collected from rural/isolated areas are sent to laboratories in major cities, there are delays in delivering results due to limited standard equipment and expertise. This situation also impacts the delay in commencing optimal treatment [50, 51].

Apart from facility limitations, a study in Pakistan indicated a lack of awareness among healthcare professionals regarding colorectal cancer symptoms. For instance, many doctors often overlook the significance of blood in stool, especially in individuals older than 50 years, requiring further investigation. Complaints about blood in the stool cannot simply be associated with hemorrhoids and disregarded. Additionally, in medical history-taking, the specific risk factors for colorectal cancer, particularly genetic aspects, are frequently underexplored. First-degree family members of patients with colorectal cancer are seldom informed about their higher risk for this malignancy, necessitating screening as per indications [52].

4. Challenges in the CRC screening in developing countries

Until now, the recommended population-based CRC screening option is a stool test, such as FOBT/gFOBT and the FIT/iFOBT immunochemical examination which can be used to detect small amounts of blood in stool samples from asymptomatic and medium-risk patients. However, in developing country settings or low-middle-income countries (LMIC), this approach is often unsuccessful due to limited resources and infrastructure [53, 54]. The following are some of the challenges in CRC screening in developing countries.

4.1 Lack of registry, poor reporting data

CRC cases are often not well recorded in cancer registries in several developing countries. This is because the process of collecting data and reporting CRC cases is not an obligation. This causes epidemiological data including incidence, mortality, and screening numbers of CRC patients to be often limited [55]. This condition then leads to the problem of CRC being underrepresented as a health problem and leading to low funding allocated by the government for CRC treatment programs [53, 56].

In several developing countries with a low incidence of CRC, screening programs are often not a priority for health programs. This can also be caused by underestimation of the CRC problem itself which can be caused by a lack of reliable epidemiological data [53, 56].

4.2 Lack of knowledge, awareness

The condition of society in general is less aware of CRC, CRC screening, and the urgency of early detection of CRC. The low level of public knowledge about CRC can also be caused by a lack of activities that can increase public awareness about CRC. This is in line with the public's lack of knowledge regarding the available screening method options and several CRC risk factors [53, 56]. Althobaiti and Jradi's research found that the public's low interest in screening was related to the public's low knowledge about screening options and the symptoms of CRC [57].

Furthermore, low knowledge of CRC among people in developing countries can also be caused by the low level of education in these areas it fails to form public awareness and attitudes towards the disease. Research on the elderly population in Saudi Arabia shows that education about the signs, symptoms, and risk factors of CRC has a positive impact on people's awareness and desire to undergo screening [58]. Research in China shows that people who know the choice of CRC screening methods are 6 times more likely to undergo CRC screening than people who do not know all [59].

4.3 Inadequate human resources and skills

Some CRC screening methods require experts in the field to assist in the diagnosis process. However, in developing countries, expert human resources are often limited, such as oncologists, endoscopists, gastroenterologists, and radiotherapists. This condition is also exacerbated by the low opportunities for training for health service providers so that resource development becomes limited and leads to low levels of CRC screening and management services [53, 56].

In developing countries, existing health staff often have limited knowledge and skills regarding CRC screening procedures [60]. Althobaiti's research found that medical students' knowledge of CRC risk factors and available screening methods was relatively low. This can then result in a lack of recommendations or encouragement issued by health workers to the public to carry out screening [57].

4.4 Poor infrastructure

CRC screening services require adequate equipment and health service providers, but in some developing countries, this is limited. Available screening facilities are often not widely available and require long waiting times for colonoscopy or endoscopy examinations [61]. Some screening equipment is also limited and not available in the entire network of screening facilities. In some cases, people often find it difficult to access screening facilities due to long distances and extreme terrain, especially those who live in rural areas [53, 56].

4.5 Absence of screening guideline

In several developing countries, there are often no adequate screening guidelines based on the latest recommendations. Apart from that, existing screening guidelines often do not facilitate the availability of equipment, especially in first-level health facilities, so screening targets are not optimal [53, 56].

4.6 Cost and financial issues

Countries with a low incidence of CRC often do not prioritize CRC screening programs so budgets are limited. This condition causes the development of screening programs which include the development of infrastructure, tools, human resources, and access to services to be limited [62]. Limited budgets also mean that CRC screening often requires large costs and must be borne by the patient, which reduces people's interest in screening [53, 56].

5. Recommendation or future strategies for CRC screening in developing countries

Potentially, a greater comprehension of the etiology and risk elements associated with colorectal cancer (CRC) may enhance the precision of cancer screenings and result in more favorable prognoses. Further technological developments are necessary in the coming years to improve the diagnostic sensitivity of screening tests and decrease the incidence of false negatives. Concurrently, additional non-invasive tests should be implemented to aid in increasing adherence to surveillance programs and decrease the need for invasive screening [63].

There are currently insufficient empirical findings to establish a definitive superior approach, so it is impossible to define a universally ideal screening strategy for colorectal cancer. The optimal choice is the one that is both financially feasible and to which patients can most readily conform in the long run [8, 63]. Screening for colorectal cancer (CRC) should commence at 50 years of age for at-risk populations, be tailored for patients between 76 and 85 years of age based on the presence of comorbidities, and cease for patients aged 85 years or older, or when the patient's age or general condition "a priori" precludes any treatment option [7, 63]. Fecal occult blood tests (FOBT) and fecal immunochemical tests (FIT) are economical, non-invasive, and well-tolerated fecal occult blood tests. There is substantial evidence to support conducting testing annually or every 2 years. As a recall strategy, positive test results necessitate that subjects undergo a colonoscopy to confirm or rule out the presence of a tumor [63].

6. Conclusion

Challenges to CRC screening in developing countries include insufficient infrastructure and trained personnel, limited endoscopic capacity, and a lack of individual awareness. Greater facility availability and individual awareness would help overcome barriers in CRC screening. Implementation of intake interventions must consider and respond to differences in each country's health systems, economies, and infrastructure.

Author details

Gede Eka Rusdi Antara
Faculty of Medicine, Department of Surgery, Udayana University, Denpasar, Indonesia

*Address all correspondence to: dr_rusdi@yahoo.com

References

[1] GLOBOCAN. Estimated number of new cases in 2020, worldwide, both sexes, all ages [Internet]. The Global Cancer Observatory. WHO. 2020. Available from: https://gco.iarc.fr

[2] Hossain MS, Karuniawati H, Jairoun AA, Urbi Z, Ooi DJ, John A, et al. Colorectal cancer: A review of carcinogenesis, global epidemiology, current challenges, risk factors, preventive and treatment strategies. Cancers. 2022;**14**:1732

[3] Herman AM, Hawkins AT, Misso K, Issangya C, Tarmohamed M, Mremi A, et al. Colorectal cancer in northern Tanzania: Increasing trends and late presentation present major challenges [internet]. JCO Global Oncology. 2020;**6**, **6**:375-381. Available from: https://ascopubs.org/go/authors/open-access

[4] Chalya PL, Mchembe MD, Mabula JB, Rambau PF, Jaka H, Koy M, et al. Clinicopathological patterns and challenges of management of colorectal cancer in a resource-limited setting: A Tanzanian experience [internet]. World Journal of Surgical Oncology. 2013;**11**:88. Available from: http://www.wjso.com/content/11/1/88

[5] Onyoh EF, Hsu WF, Chang LC, Lee YC, Wu MS, Chiu HM. The rise of colorectal cancer in Asia: Epidemiology, screening, and management. Current Gastroenterology Reports. 2019;**21**:36

[6] Schliemann D, Ramanathan K, Matovu N, O'Neill C, Kee F, Su TT, et al. The implementation of colorectal cancer screening interventions in low and middle-income countries: A scoping review. BMC Cancer. 2021;**21**(1):1125

[7] Lopes G, Stern MC, Temin S, Sharara AI, Cervantes A, Costas-Chavarri A, et al. Early detection for colorectal cancer: ASCO resource-stratified guideline. Journal of Global Oncology. 2019;**5**:1-22; Available from: https://ascopubs.org/go/authors/open-access

[8] Brenner H, Chen C. The colorectal cancer epidemic: Challenges and opportunities for primary, secondary and tertiary prevention. British Journal of Cancer. 2018;**119**:785-792

[9] Rawla P, Sunkara T, Barsouk A. Epidemiology of colorectal cancer: Incidence, mortality, survival, and risk factors. Przeglad Gastroenterologiczny. 2019;**14**:89-103

[10] Sawicki T, Ruszkowska M, Danielewicz A, Niedźwiedzka E, Arłukowicz T, Przybyłowicz KE. A review of colorectal cancer in terms of epidemiology, risk factors, development, symptoms and diagnosis. Cancers. 2021;**13**:2025

[11] Rafiemanesh H, Mohammadian-Hafshejani A, Ghoncheh M, Sepehri Z, Shamlou R, Salehiniya H, et al. Incidence and mortality of colorectal cancer and relationships with the human development index across the world. Asian Pacific Journal of Cancer Prevention. 2016;**17**(5):2465-2473

[12] Bishehsari F, Mahdavinia M, Vacca M, Malekzadeh R, Mariani-Costantini R. Epidemiological transition of colorectal cancer in developing countries: Environmental factors, molecular pathways, and opportunities for prevention. World Journal of Gastroenterology. 2014;**20**(20):6055-6072

[13] Safiri S, Sepanlou SG, Ikuta KS, Bisignano C, Salimzadeh H, Delavari A,

et al. The global, regional, and national burden of colorectal cancer and its attributable risk factors in 195 countries and territories, 1990-2017: A systematic analysis for the global burden of disease study 2017. The Lancet Gastroenterology & Hepatology. 2019;**4**(12):913-933

[14] Awedew AF, Asefa Z, Belay WB. Burden and trend of colorectal cancer in 54 countries of Africa 2010-2019: A systematic examination for global burden of disease. BMC Gastroenterology. 2022;**22**(1):204

[15] Graham A, Adeloye D, Grant L, Theodoratou E, Campbell H. Estimating the incidence of colorectal cancer in sub-Saharan Africa: A systematic analysis. Journal of Global Health. 2012;**2**(2):020404

[16] Xi Y, Xu P. Global colorectal cancer burden in 2020 and projections to 2040. Translational Oncology. 2021;**14**:101174

[17] Mattiuzzi C, Sanchis-Gomar F, Lippi G. Concise update on colorectal cancer epidemiology. Annals of Translational Medicine. 2019;7(21):609-609

[18] American Cancer Society. American Cancer Society Guideline for Colorectal Cancer Screening [Internet]. USA: American Cancer Society; 2020. Available from: https://www.cancer.org/cancer/types/ colon-rectal-cancer/detection-diagnosisstaging/acs-recommendations.html

[19] Kemenkes RI. Pedoman Nasional Pelayanan Kedokteran Tata Laksana Kanker Kolorektal. Jakarta: Kementerian Kesehatan Republik Indonesia; 2018

[20] Nyitray AG, D'Souza G, Stier EA, Clifford G, Chiao EY. The utility of digital anal rectal examinations in a public health screening program for anal cancer. Journal of Lower Genital Tract Disease. 2020;**24**(2):192

[21] Hillman RJ, Berry-Lawhorn JM, Ong JJ, Cuming T, Nathan M, Goldstone S, et al. International anal neoplasia society guidelines for the practice of digital anal rectal examination. Journal of Lower Genital Tract Disease. 2019;**23**(2):138-146

[22] Tanaka A, Sadahiro S, Suzuki T, Okada K, Saito G. Comparisons of rigid proctoscopy, flexible colonoscopy, and digital rectal examination for determining the localization of rectal cancers. Diseases of the Colon and Rectum. 2018;**61**(2):202-206

[23] Santare D, Kojalo I, Huttunen T, Rikacovs S, Rucevskis P, Boka V, et al. Improving uptake of screening for colorectal cancer: A study on invitation strategies and different test kit use. European Journal of Gastroenterology & Hepatology. 2015;**27**(5):536

[24] Khakimov N, Khasanova G, Ershova K, Gibadullina L, Vetkina T, Lobisheva G, et al. Screening for colon cancer: A test for occult blood. International Journal of Risk & Safety in Medicine. 2015;**27**(s1):S110-S111

[25] Kościelniak-Merak B, Radosavljević B, Zając A, Tomasik PJ. Faecal occult blood point-of-care tests. Journal of Gastrointestinal Cancer. 2018;**49**:402-405

[26] Benton SC, Seaman HE, Halloran SP. Faecal occult blood testing for colorectal cancer screening: The past or the future. Current Gastroenterology Reports. 2015;**17**(2):7

[27] Wang H-Y, Lin T-W, Chiu SY-H, Lin W-Y, Huang S-B, Hsieh JC-H, et al. Novel toilet paper–based point-of-care test for the rapid detection of fecal occult

blood: Instrument validation study. Journal of Medical Internet Research. 2020;**22**(8):e20261

[28] Rex DK, Boland CR, Dominitz JA, Giardiello FM, Johnson DA, Kaltenbach T, et al. Colorectal cancer screening: Recommendations for physicians and patients from the U.S. multi-society task force on colorectal cancer. Gastroenterology. 2017;**153**(1):307-323

[29] Wolf AMD, Fontham ETH, Church TR, Flowers CR, Guerra CE, LaMonte SJ, et al. Colorectal cancer screening for average-risk adults: 2018 guideline update from the American Cancer Society. CA: a Cancer Journal for Clinicians. 2018;**68**(4):250-281

[30] Li D. Recent advances in colorectal cancer screening. Chronic Diseases and Translational Medicine. 2018;**4**:139-147

[31] Nishihara R, Wu K, Lochhead P, Morikawa T, Liao X, Qian ZR, et al. Long-term colorectal-cancer incidence and mortality after lower endoscopy. New England Journal of Medicine. 2013;**369**(12):1095-1105

[32] Reumkens A, Rondagh EJA, Bakker CM, Winkens B, Masclee AAM, Sanduleanu S. Post-colonoscopy complications: A systematic review, time trends, and meta-analysis of population-based studies. American Journal of Gastroenterology. 2016;**111**:1092-1101

[33] Holme Ø, Løberg M, Kalager M, Bretthauer M, Hernán MA, Aas E, et al. Effect of flexible sigmoidoscopy screening on colorectal cancer incidence and mortality: A randomized clinical trial. Journal of the American Medical Association. 2014;**312**(6):606-615

[34] Atkin W, Wooldrage K, Parkin DM, Kralj-Hans I, MacRae E, Shah U, et al. Long term effects of once-only flexible sigmoidoscopy screening after 17 years of follow-up: The UK flexible sigmoidoscopy screening randomised controlled trial. The Lancet. 2017;**389**(10076):1299-1311

[35] Bibbins-Domingo K, Grossman DC, Curry SJ, Davidson KW, Epling JW, García FAR, et al. Screening for colorectal cancer: US preventive services task force recommendation statement. JAMA - Journal of the American Medical Association. 2016;**315**(23):2564-2575

[36] Imperiale TF, Ransohoff DF, Itzkowitz SH, Levin TR, Lavin P, Lidgard GP, et al. Multitarget stool DNA testing for colorectal-cancer screening. New England Journal of Medicine. 2014;**370**(14):1287-1297

[37] Halligan S, Wooldrage K, Dadswell E, Kralj-Hans I, Von Wagner C, Edwards R, et al. Computed tomographic colonography versus barium enema for diagnosis of colorectal cancer or large polyps in symptomatic patients (SIGGAR): A multicentre randomised trial. The Lancet. 2013;**381**(9873):1185-1193

[38] Lin JS, Piper MA, Perdue LA, Rutter CM, Webber EM, O'Connor E, et al. Screening for colorectal cancer: Updated evidence report and systematic review for the US preventive services task force. JAMA - Journal of the American Medical Association. 2016;**315**(23):2576-2594

[39] Shaukat A, Levin TR. Current and future colorectal cancer screening strategies. Nature Reviews Gastroenterology and Hepatology. Nature Research. 2022;**19**:521-531

[40] Ijspeert JEG, Tutein Nolthenius CJ, Kuipers EJ, Van Leerdam ME, Nio CY,

Thomeer MGJ, et al. CT-Colonography vs. colonoscopy for detection of high-risk sessile serrated polyps. American Journal of Gastroenterology. 2016;**111**(4):516-522

[41] Babayan A, Pantel K. Advances in liquid biopsy approaches for early detection and monitoring of cancer. Genome Medicine. 2018;**10**:21

[42] Church TR, Wandell M, Lofton-Day C, Mongin SJ, Burger M, Payne SR, et al. Prospective evaluation of methylated SEPT9 in plasma for detection of asymptomatic colorectal cancer. Gut. 2014;**63**(2):317-325

[43] Parikh RB, Prasad V. Blood-based screening for colon cancer a disruptive innovation or simply a disruption? Journal of the American Medical Association. 2016;**315**:2519-2520. Available from: http://jama.jamanetwork.com/

[44] Simon K. Colorectal cancer development and advances in screening. In: Clinical Interventions in Aging. Vol. 11. [Internet]. UK: Dove Medical Press Ltd; 2016. pp. 967-976. Available from: https://www.dovepress.com/

[45] Zhang M, He Y, Zhang X, Zhang M, Kong L. A pooled analysis of the diagnostic efficacy of plasmic methylated septin-9 as a novel biomarker for colorectal cancer. Biomedical Reports. 2017;7:353-360

[46] Unger-Saldaña K, Saldaña-Tellez M, Potter MB, Van Loon K, Allen-Leigh B, Lajous M. Barriers and facilitators for colorectal cancer screening in a low-income urban community in Mexico City. Implementation Science Communications. 2020;**1**(1):64

[47] Jiao YF, Cheng ZY, Gao Y, Yu CT, Jiang HS, Wang TL, et al. Development, quality, and influencing factors of colonoscopy in China: Results from the national census in 2013 and 2020. Frontiers in Oncology. 2023;**13**:1276520

[48] Makmun D. Present status of endoscopy, therapeutic endoscopy and the endoscopy training system in Indonesia. Digestive Endoscopy. 2014;**26**:2-9

[49] Kuga R, Facanali Junior MR, ELA DA. Quality indicators in colonoscopy: Observational study in a supplementary health system. Acta Cirúrgica Brasileira. 2022;**37**(11):e371106

[50] Ngoya PS, Muhogora WE, Pitcher RD. Defining the diagnostic divide: An analysis of registered radiological equipment resources in a low-income African country. Pan African Medical Journal. 2016;**25**:99

[51] Khan SZ, Lengyel CG. Challenges in the management of colorectal cancer in low- and middle-income countries. Cancer Treatment and Research Communications. 2023;**35**:100705

[52] Ahmed F. Barriers to colorectal cancer screening in the developing world: The view from Pakistan. World Journal of Gastrointestinal Pharmacology and Therapeutics. 2013;**4**(4):83

[53] Schliemann D, Ramanathan K, Matovu N, O'Neill C, Kee F, Su TT, et al. The implementation of colorectal cancer screening interventions in low-and middle-income countries: A scoping review. BMC Cancer. 2021;**21**(1):1125

[54] Wilson LAM, Browne S, Barnes J, El Hoyek N, Helmueller L, Janeiro MJ, et al. Opportunities and challenges in screening for colorectal cancer. Population Health Management. 2023;**26**(4):246-253

[55] Gupta S, Sussman DA, Doubeni CA, Anderson DS, Day L, Deshpande AR,

et al. Challenges and possible solutions to colorectal cancer screening for the underserved. Journal of the National Cancer Institute. 2014;**106**:dju032

[56] Hatamian S, Hadavandsiri F, Momenimovahed Z, Salehiniya H. Barriers and facilitators of colorectal cancer screening in Asia. Ecancermedicalscience. 2021;**15**:1285

[57] Althobaiti A, Jradi H. Knowledge, attitude, and perceived barriers regarding colorectal cancer screening practices and risk factors among medical students in Saudi Arabia. BMC Medical Education. 2019;**19**(1):421

[58] Galal YS, Amin TT, Alarfaj AK, Almulhim AA, Aljughaiman AA, Almulla AK, et al. Colon cancer among older saudis: Awareness of risk factors and early signs, and perceived barriers to screening. Asian Pacific Journal of Cancer Prevention. 2016;**17**(4):1837-1846

[59] Bai Y, Wong CL, He X, Wang C, So WKW. Effectiveness of tailored communication intervention in increasing colonoscopy screening rates amongst first-degree relatives of individuals with colorectal cancer: A systematic review and meta-analysis. International Journal of Nursing Studies. 2020;**101**:103397

[60] Quintero E, Hassan C, Senore C, Saito Y. Progress and challenges in colorectal cancer screening. Gastroenterology Research and Practice. 2012;**2012**:846985

[61] Liles EG, Schneider JL, Feldstein AC, Mosen DM, Perrin N, Rosales AG, et al. Implementation challenges and successes of a population-based colorectal cancer screening program: A qualitative study of stakeholder perspectives. Implementation Science. 2015;**10**(1):41

[62] Lu CH, Bin Dai M. Colorectal cancer screening in China: Status, challenges, and prospects-China [internet]. China CDC Weekly. 2022;**4**(15):322-328. Available from: https://gco.iarc.fr/

[63] Maida M, Macaluso FS, Ianiro G, Mangiola F, Sinagra E, Hold G, et al. Screening of colorectal cancer: Present and future. Expert Review of Anticancer Therapy. 2017;**17**:1131-1146

Chapter 2

Biomarkers as a Therapeutic Approach in Colorectal Carcinoma

Rustam Effendi-YS, Amido Rey and Imelda Rey

Abstract

This review highlights the most promising biomarker tests of tumor tissue from colonoscopy biopsy for more individualized therapeutic approaches to patients with colorectal carcinoma (CRC). Biomarkers are a key tool in early detection, survival, and predicting treatment response and prognostic value. The tests can help doctors to select a specific CRC treatment and targeted therapy. CRC is the third most common cancer diagnosed, and the second leading cause of cancer-related deaths worldwide, despite the progress made in detection and management through surgery, chemotherapy, radiotherapy, and immunotherapy. With a population totaling 273,523,621 people, Indonesia has estimated 396,914 new cases of all cancer and 234,511 cancer-related deaths. Among those cancer cases, estimated 34,189 new CRC cases and 17,786 CRC deaths occurred in 2020. Most of CRC cases were located in the rectum compared to those in the distal colon or proximal colon. CRC is a heterogeneous cancer. Its therapeutic approaches vary, depending on the tumor location (proximal, distal colon, or rectum), clinical signs and symptoms, staging and biomarkers such as KRAS and NRAS, BRAF V600E, MSI high (dMMR), CIN, HER2-amplified, PD-1, CTLA-4, MEK, and NTRK gene fusion-positive. CSCs and other biomarkers are being developed and remain under investigation.

Keywords: colorectal carcinoma, tumor locations, biomarkers, systemic therapy, targeted therapy

1. Introduction

Colorectal cancer (CRC) is the third most common cancer and the second leading cause of cancer deaths among all cancers worldwide. There were an estimated of 1,931,590 new CRC cases (10% of an estimated 19.3 million new cases of all cancers), and 915,880 CRC deaths (9.2% of all cancer deaths) worldwide in 2020. Indonesia, with a total population of 273,523,621, estimatedly has 396,914 new cancer cases and 234,511 cancer-related deaths. Among those cancer cases, an estimated of 34,189 new CRC cases and 17,786 CRC deaths occurred in 2020 [1–3]. A total of 74.6% of CRC cases were found in the rectum, whereas those found in the distal colon and the proximal colon were 18.8% and 6.6% respectively [1].

Rising treatment costs for colorectal cancer, which is significantly higher than the average increase in health costs, present a considerable concern for policy makers.

These CRC costs translate to increasing economic burden for Asia and Indonesia, not unlike what has been happening in Western countries [4].

A better understanding of the molecular pathways in the carcinogenesis of CRC influenced by the genetic and epigenetic changes, and the interactions between microenvironment and germline factors, has helped develop the current management of CRC patients. Doctors can choose a specific course of CRC treatment based on the biomarker tests of tumor tissue from a colonoscopy biopsy, and they can use the tests to determine diagnostic and prognostic value, predictive factors, and targeted therapy. Examining KRAS, BRAF, and microsatellite instability (MSI) is crucial in order to establish an appropriate therapy for advanced or metastatic CRC [1, 5, 6].

There has been a published study on CRC biomarkers based on the three locations [7, 8]. This study reported that there were differences in the characteristics of chromosome instability (CIN), mismatch repair (MMR), and microsatellite instability (MSI) found in the different locations (proximal colon, distal colon, and rectum) [7, 8]. The MLH1 protein expression negative was prominent in proximal colon cancer, MSH6 in distal and rectal cancer, and APC in distal colon cancer, respectively. The MSI-H proportion was more likely to occur in proximal rather than in distal or rectal cancer. These findings suggest that the CRC in each location has its own specific molecular characteristics i.e., unique underlying carcinogenic pathways or molecular backgrounds [6–8]. More than 50% of CRC patients will develop metastasis, and approximately 25% of them present with metastasis at initial diagnosis [1, 6, 8].

CRC is a heterogeneous cancer, and the location of the tumor, clinical symptoms, CRC stage, and biomarkers play a significant role in determining the therapeutic approaches [1, 4, 7, 8].

There are two types of screening tests to detect CRC early: the non-invasive test by examining patient's stool (including gFOBT, FIT, and sDNA tests), and the invasive colonoscopy. When the non-invasive tests yield a positive result, the patient must then undergo a colonoscopy to confirm the diagnosis [4, 9].

Inherited/familial CRC is caused by germline mutations, while sporadic CRC is caused by somatic mutations and is not associated with family history. Genetic and epigenetic changes are involved in the formation of CRC. In the multistep genetic model for colorectal carcinogenesis, there are three major pathways involved in the genetic instability of CRC and its pathogenesis, namely chromosomal instability (CIN), microsatellite instability (MSI), and CpG island methylator phenotype (CIMP) pathways. Adenomatous polyps, sessile serrated lesions and traditional serrated adenomas can grow into colorectal cancer. In the serrated pathway, RAS and RAF mutations were found, as well as disturbances in the Wnt signaling pathway, and CpG island methylation [10–13].

Biomarker tests affect therapeutic strategies chosen for colorectal cancer patients. Targeted therapies are recommended for advanced or mCRC patients with mutated KRAS/NRAS/BRAF or wild-type tumors, HER2-amplified tumors, and those with NTRK gene fusion-positive, whereas those with MSI-High (dMMR) status are given immunotherapy. Utilizing biomarkers in clinical settings is ever progressing and remains a challenge for more in-depth study [1, 6, 8, 11, 12].

2. Diagnostic approach

The clinical signs and symptoms presented by CRC patients are related to the tumor location, size, and CRC stage [1, 6–8]. It is possible for patients to exhibit no symptoms in the early stages. The frequently reported symptoms are changes in bowel habit, such as diarrhea, constipation or change in the stool consistency, bloody (bright red) stool (hematochezia), stomach pain/cramps, bloating, feeling full, fatigue, or exhaustion, lower appetite, unexplained iron deficiency anemia, or weight loss. Physical examination is focused on finding abdominal mass, especially at the right and left iliac fossa, right upper abdomen, as well as finding possible metastatic lesions, enlarged lymph nodes, hepatomegaly, etc. In addition, a digital rectal examination (DRE) is also needed.

Patients with proximal colon cancer, especially at the cecum may have abdominal mass, particularly at the right iliac fossa, while patients with sigmoid cancer will have palpable mass at the left iliac fossa. Common signs and symptoms of emergencies due to complications of CRC should be examined, such as peritonitis from perforation, or obstruction. Other signs, such as jaundice, hepatomegaly, and ascites may occur with liver metastases [1, 11–13].

2.1 Colonoscopy and biopsy

The gold standard tools for diagnosing CRC are colonoscopy and tumor biopsy. They are also useful preventive methods through screening and removing polyps or premalignant lesions in the colorectal. The popular endoscopic techniques to remove colon polyps or precancer growths are polypectomy, endoscopic mucosal resection (EMR), or endoscopic submucosal dissection (ESD) [1, 9, 10, 13].

The currently available non-invasive screening tools are not sensitive enough to detect pre-cancerous lesions and early-stage CRC. As such, colonoscopy is still required to establish early CRC in patients [5].

2.2 Biomarker tests of tumor tissue biopsy

To determine the histology and examine the biomarkers of the tumor, first, a specimen of fresh tissue from colonoscopy biopsy is fixated using 10% formaldehyde buffering solution and made into paraffin blocks known as formalin-fixed and paraffin-embedded tissues (FFPET). Then a special staining process i.e., hematoxylin and eosin staining (H&E) is conducted to determine the histology of the tumor, and immunohistochemistry (IHC) test to examine biomarker tests, to detect evidence of chromosome instability (CIN) such as adenomatous polyposis coli (APC) protein expression, MMR defect, MSI status, KRAS, BRAF v600E mutation status. PCR test is also used for the detection of MSI and CpG island methylation phenotype (CIMP) [1, 6, 8, 11, 12].

2.3 Laboratory examination

The common laboratory examinations required are complete blood count, urinalysis, serum chemistries e.g., hepatic function panel, kidney function tests, etc. Another recommended test before and after surgery is carcinoembryonic antigen (CEA), which may be needed every 6 months if cancer recurrence is suspected [1, 12].

2.4 CT scan or MRI

To determine the condition of the disease and detect metastases in CRC patients, several examinations such as CT scanning of the chest, CT scanning of the abdomen, and pelvis, and especially MRI or transrectal USG (TRUS) for rectal cancer, are necessary. These examinations provide information about the staging of colorectal cancer patients [1, 11, 12].

3. Treatment

There are several factors to consider in the treatment of CRC patients. They are the stage of the disease according to TNM classification, the tumor location (proximal colon, distal colon, or rectum), clinical signs, intestinal obstruction, biomarker test results, patient's general physical condition, and the treatment purpose (curative or palliative). The treatment options include surgery (surgical resection, excision), and systemic therapy consisting of chemotherapy, targeted therapy, and immunotherapy. Cancer stage, circumferential resection margin, lymph-vascular invasion, perineural invasion, and genotyping are considered as well to decide on the need for and the type of adjuvant therapy. Therapeutic management is ideally a multidisciplinary approach consisting of accurate diagnosis, cutting-edge surgical technique, biomarker tests, optimal selection of drugs/procedure, and informed consent [5, 11–16].

3.1 Surgery

The main treatment for CRC is surgery limited to the colon or rectum. In the early stage of CRC, removing cancerous tissues including tumors and lymph nodes is expected to prevent the cancer from spreading. In the later stages, however, surgery cannot stop the growth or spreading. Available options for stage 4 CRC patients are: blockage-removal surgery, radiation, or chemotherapy to reduce the tumor size, pain relief, treatment to manage the side effects of medication, and counseling [12–15].

3.2 Systemic therapy

Localized and advanced CRC can be treated by systemic therapy including chemotherapy, targeted therapy, immunotherapy, and some recent therapies, or a newly developed therapy.

The goal of these therapies is to reduce the size of the tumor/metastases to a resectable status, thus increasing a patient's chance of progression-free survival. *Chemotherapy* works by destroying cancerous cells throughout the body. It is useful to help shrink the tumor before surgery and relieve symptoms in the advanced stages. However, since chemotherapy targets both healthy and cancerous cells, it can have extensive negative effects or adverse effects on a patient's body.

Targeted therapy targets specific protein molecules in order to prevent/slow down the cancer cells' growth. The adverse effects are usually less severe than those of chemotherapy because these drugs only target specific cells. Immunotherapy block the cancer cells' ability that stop the immune system, and is recommended for advanced CRC show MSI-high. Numerous newly developed therapies and biomarkers are available and reviewed in this article [1, 12–17].

4. Biomarkers in CRC

Biomarkers tests serve as a guide to cancer therapy and they can also be used as a screening test to detect the disease early. The tests can be categorized into three:

diagnostic, prognostic, and predictive. In each different stage of CRC, biomarkers remain functional to evaluate the disease progression, recurrence, as well as to decide on the effective and personalized treatment for patients [5, 18–22]. Early detection of CRC is crucial, and there are two main methods of screening tests: non-invasive and invasive. Non-invasive method examines patient's stool by conducting tests such as gFOBT, fecal immunochemical test (FIT), and stool DNA tests (sDNA); while invasive methods is the form of colonoscopy. Using FIT and sDNA to screen for advanced precancerous lesions has low sensitivities, and, in terms of detecting polyps with high-grade dysplasia, and sessile serrated polyps >1 cm, both tests also have low abilities. Therefore, due to the limitations/insensitivities of non-invasive screening tests, they must be followed up by colonoscopy to confirm the diagnosis [1, 4, 5, 9].

Colorectal cancer can be categorized as one of these groups: sporadic, familial, and hereditary CRC. Sporadic CRC is the most frequently found type (70–80%). It originates from somatic mutations and is not related to family history. The progression to CRC is explained as the result of various genetic and epigenetic changes accumulated overtime [1, 7, 8, 11, 21].

Chromosomal instability (CIN) leads to mutations or loss of protein expression of tumor suppressor genes, e.g., APC, P53, SMAD4, etc. And the mutation of these tumor suppressor genes such as APC, p53, p27, and MSI-H, LOH 18q, DNA hypermethylationwith the activation of oncogenes, including KRAS,NRAS,BRAF, EGFR (Erb-B1), Erb-B2, can assist cancer growth or promote cancer cell survival and suppress apoptosis.

Some biomarkers are based on the mutational status of tumor suppressor genes or oncogenes known to be important in carcinogenesis of CRC, or based on defects in DNA MMR (dMMR), MSI status, and CpG Island methylator phenotype methylation.

4.1 RAS mutation

There are three oncogenes of the RAS oncogene family, namely Kirsten rat sarcoma (KRAS), Neuroblastoma (NRAS), and Harvey rat sarcoma oncogene homolog (HRAS). RAS stimulates various signaling pathways, including the RAS-RAF-MEK-ERK and the phosphatidylinositol 3-kinase (PI3K) pathways [17].

CIN trigger CRC via TSG (e.g., APC, TP53) loss or mutation and the activation of oncogenes such as KRAS genes [6]. In many cases KRAS mutations occur in codon 12 of exon 2 [6].

In terms of clinical purpose, the recommended clinical guideline is to extend the KRAS mutation testing in CRC patients to include KRAS and NRAS in exon 2 (codons 12 and 13), exon 3 (codon 59 and 61), and exon 4 (codon 117 and 146) [23]. KRAS mutation indicates lack of/poor response to anti-EGFR therapy using cetuximab and panitumumab. So anti-EGFR therapy is not the treatment suggested for patients whose tumor has a KRAS mutation [6]. Testing for KRAS is recommended for stage IV patients and any stage of recurrence. NRAS testing is typically put forward for stage IV patients and stage III recurrence. Patients with wild-type NRAS may have a positive reaction to certain treatment plans that include EGFR inhibitors [19].

4.2 BRAF mutations

Mutation in BRAF appears about 12% in all CRC patients; in addition, BRAF and KRAS mutations are mutually exclusive [6]. When KRAS mutation is not found, then it is suggested to test for BRAF [6]. BRAF mutation is strongly correlated with

MSI-H/dMMR status. In the cases of sporadic CRC, BRAF mutation is present in 60% of MSI-H tumors but only 5–10% in MSS tumors. This correlation distinguishes sporadic MSI-H/dMMR from Lynch syndrome because the BRAFV600E mutation excludes Lynch syndrome but is related to CRC patients. The presence of BRAFV600E mutation has a negative prognosis for stage II and III CRC [17]. The BRAF proto-oncogene works via the RAS-RAF-MEK-ERK pathway regulating cell transcription. In comparison to wild-type BRAF, the BRAFV600E mutation generally means lower survival rate i.e., lower progression-free and up to 50% worse overall survival rates [5].

Patients with BRAF mutation may not respond to EGFR-inhibitor drugs (cetuximab and panitumumab); there may be a poorer prognosis, and the use of standard chemotherapy may not yield the expected good results. BRAF testing is commonly used for stage IV patients, which can be simultaneously done with NRAS and KRAS tests [19, 23]. If found, BRAFV600E indicates a particularly aggressive cancer that needs to be treated aggressively. Approximately 20% of patients with BRAF V600E-mutated mCRC also have MSI-H. Just like any other patients with MSI-H, these patients can respond to checkpoint inhibitors such as nivolumab and pembrolizumab [24].

A number of signaling pathways involved in the initiation, progression, and migration of CRC, is an ideal sites for targeted therapy such as Wnt/β catenin, Notch, Hedgehog, and TGF-β (transforming growth factor-β)/SMAD, as well as those capable of activating signaling cascades, such as phosphatidylinositol 3-kinase (PI3K)/AKT or RAS/RAF.

The EGFR pathway belongs to the ErbB/HER family that, once activated, will trigger various downstream intracellular signaling pathways, including RAS/RAF/MEK/ERK, PI3K/AKT, and JAK/STAT3 (Janus kinase/signal transducer and transcription activator), to manage cell growth, survival and migration [25].

4.3 The carcinoembryonic antigen (CEA)

CEA, a high molecular weight glycoprotein, is used as a biomarker to foresee early recurrence in post-surgical patients. It is useful as a prognostic biomarker that may change thresholds for further study of recurring cancers and higher chance of early intervention [5]. To determine the presence of CRC post-operative recurrence, CEA examination is performed before and after surgery [13].

4.4 MSI status and d-MMR

MSI is a clonal change in the number of repeated DNA nucleotide units in microsatellites; it is also known as a change in the length of a simple repeated nucleotide sequence [7, 8].

MSI occurs as a result of MMR deficiency caused by the inactivity of one (or more) of the four MMR genes. A high MSI status (MSI-H) or deficient MMR (d-MMR) can be established through IHC test or PCR examination. In essence, MSI can be defined as the loss of protein expression of MLH1, MSH2, MSH6, and PMS2 found upon immunohistochemical examination. PCR test using five microsatellite markers (Bethesda panel) i.e., D2S123, D5S346, D17S250, BAT25, and BAT26, can be used to check MSI level. If the results show instability in two or more microsatellite markers, it is categorized as MSI-H [1, 7, 8, 11]; and if no instability found, it means a stable microsatellite (MSS) also known as a proficient MMR (p-MMR) [21].

Around 15% of all CRC cases possess significant defects in d-MMR and the tumor tissues show MSI-H. Patients with MSI-H have a better prognosis in terms of longer overall survival and lower metastatic rate, but the tumors are more resistant to adjuvant chemotherapy such as 5-fluorouracil (5-FU) [23].

MSI status, as a predictive biomarker, is beneficial to assess mCRC patients' response to the treatment of anti-programmed cell death 1 (PD-1) checkpoint inhibitor pembrolizumab, since pembrolizumab is known to be effective only in mCRC patients with high MSI status [23].

MSI status or MMR test is a key tool and should be conducted with all CRC patients for the following reasons: (a) it is a universal screening test for Lynch syndrome (HNPCC) which is the most common cause of inherited CRC, (b) d-MMR status is well known to be indicative of a better prognosis, especially for stage II CRC patients, as is MSI-H, (c) d-MMR status is a strong negative predictive biomarker of 5-fluorouracil efficacy in stage II CRC patients, (d) in the case of mCRC, MSI-H/d-MMR status is a strong positive factor for predicting check point inhibitor (CPI) response [17]. Overall, biomarkers tests for measuring the status of MMR/MSI, and RAS/BRAF mutation are necessary to evaluate the ideal first-line therapeutic strategy.

4.5 Deficient mismatch repair (d-MMR)

d-MMR accounts for 15% of all CRC. It is observed more frequently in the early—rather than the late—stage of the disease. Loss of the MMR protein expression that can indicate deficient DNA mismatch repair (d-MMR) status can be found by doing immune histochemistry (IHC); similarly, MSI status can be determined via PCR. Because these two tests give fairly high matching results, IHC test is first performed to check MMR status. In case the finding from the IHC test is inconclusive, further test like PCR or next-generation sequencing (NGS-based assay) is recommended. MSI-H/d-MMR mCRC are more frequently right-sided and poorly differentiated and correlate more often with *BRAF* mutations [19].

5. Therapeutic approach

5.1 Current chemotherapy

Currently, available chemotherapy utilizes both single-agent and multiple-agent regiments.

The single-agent program mainly uses fluoropyrimidine (5-FU), while the multiple-agent contains one or several drugs including oxaliplatin (OX), Irinotecan (IRI), and capecitabine (CAP or XELODA or XEL). The common combinations of drugs regimens today are: FOLFOX (5-FU + OX), FOLFIRI (5-FU + IRI), XELOX or CAPOX (CAP +OX), and CAPIRI [25]. But it is worth mentioning that 5-FU is connected to toxicity and reduced clinical response in patients who have high MSI status and dihydropyrimidine dehydrogenase (DPYD) deficiency [5].

5.2 Targeted therapy

a. Anti-EGFR cetuximab and panitumumab are recommended for KRAS/NRAS/BRAF wild-type tumors.

b. Bevacizumab: anti vascular endothelial growth factor (m-Ab anti VEGFR).

c. Ramucirumab (anti VEGFR-2) acts as antineoplastic agent and direct VEGFR2 antagonist.

d. Regorafenib (multi-kinase inhibitor) blocks kinases similar to Sorafenib, but Regorafenib has more activity against VEGFR.

e. Aflibercept (recombinant fusion protein blocking VEGF A/B). It is an injection type within a class of vascular endothelial growth factor-A (VEGF-A) medications. The combination of Zif-aflibercept (a VEGF inhibitor) and FOLFIRI is stipulated to treat patients with metastatic CRC which resistant to oxaliplatin or have progressed following an oxaliplatin regimen.

(*b, c, d, and e*: recommendations for *KRAS/NRAS/BRAF mutated tumors*) [26].

5.3 Immunotherapy (recommendations for: MSI-High tumors)

The recommended immunotherapy involves Pembrolizumab (m-Ab anti PD-1), Nivolumab (anti-PD-1), and Iplimumab (anti-CTLA-4). The use of Nivolumab and Iplimumab has shown benefits in MSI-High and d-MMR genotypes patients [5, 26].

5.4 Newly developed therapies

a. For BRAFV600E mutated tumors: Vemurafenib (BRAF inhibitors), Dabrafenib (BRAF inhibitors), Encorafenib (BRAF inhibitors); Trametinib (MEK inhibitors); Binimetinib (MEK inhibitors).

b. For HER2 amplified tumors: Trastuzumab (m-Ab anti HER2), Pertuzumab (m-Ab anti HER2); Lapatinib (Dual HER2/EGFR inhibitors).

c. For NTRK gene-fusion positive tumors: Larotrectinib (TRK inhibitors); Entrectinib (TRK-inhibitors) [5, 17, 18, 26].

Glossary terms:

- MAPK: mitogen-activated protein kinase.
- MEK: mitogen-activated extracellular signal-related kinase.
- CTL-4: cytotoxic T lymphocyte-associated antigen-4.
- PD-1: programmed cell death receptor-1.
- TRK: tropomyosin receptor kinase.
- NTRK: neurotrophic tropomyosin kinase.

6. Other biomarkers used in therapeutic approach

The fact that KRAS, NRAS, BRAF, and MSI status is advocated in the evaluation of treatment response and the outcome prediction of CRC signifies the need to develop more biomarkers. In addition, several other categories of biomarkers have also shown useful potential in CRC therapeutic approach such as PD-1, CTLA-4, mitogen-activated extracellular signal-related kinase (MEK), HER2, TRK gene fusion, etc. Chemo and radio resistance that lead failure in treating primary and mCRC patients has pushed the research for the applicability of personalized medicine [27]. Another area needing further research and investigation is the use of stem cells (SCs) and cancer stem cells (CSCs) markers to develop a treatment plan; this is because CR-CSCs show an ability to self-renew and to differentiate themselves which contributes to multiple tumor malignancies e.g., recurrence, metastasis, heterogeneity, multidrug resistance, and radiation resistance [26, 28]. The use of stem cells (SCs) and cancer stem cells (CSCs) markers in such a treatment approach are necessary and further research on CR-CSCs markers are greatly needed and remains under investigation [5, 27–29].

6.1 Immune checkpoint: programmed cell death protein 1 (PD-1)

Immune system sustains the body's self-tolerance through check points such as programmed cell death protein 1 (PD1) expressed on T-cells. The attachment of ligands (programmed death ligand 1 [PD-L1] and PDL2) to programmed cell death protein 1 (PD1) brings the downregulation of effector functions. Conversely, upregulation of PD-1/PD-L1 is the mechanism that hides cancer cells from immune response which serves as the basis of the development of immunotherapy use in cancer treatment. Although immune checkpoint inhibition has seen some recent successes in many cancer treatments, it benefits only 3–7% of mCRC patients with d-MMR proteins/MSI-H [24].

PD-L1 expression is potentially useful in predicting patient's response to pembrolizumab due to the relationship between high PD-L1 expression and MSI-H status [23]. Also, neoadjuvant CPI demonstrates favorable results in treating patients with nonmetastatic CRC and MSI-H status [17]. These patients usually present poorly differentiated proximal tumors with numerous tumor-inflitrating lymphocytes, and the chance for survival is higher during the early stage (stage II). Pembrolizumab (anti-PD-1) and nivolumab (anti-PD-1) are IgG4 m-Abs that bind to PD-1, and they are FDA-approved as the subsequent-line of treatment of d-MMR or MSI-H mCRC [24].

In the case of mCRC, the anti-programmed cell death receptor-1 agents or anti-PD1 (Nivolumab) and anti CTLA-4 (Ipilimumab) have been advantageous in MSI-High tumors and mismatch repair deficient genotypes, thus being acknowledged for patients progressing on first-line chemotherapy [5].

6.2 Human epidermal growth factor receptor 2 (HER2, Erb-B2)

The human epidermal growth factor2 (HER2) is a proto-oncogene located on chromosome 17q21 that encodes for a transmembrane glycoprotein receptor with tyrosine kinase activity [30]. HER2 alterations e.g., somatic mutations and amplifications are present only in 3–5% metastatic colorectal cancer patients. HER2 was first assessed as a biomarker of resistance to anti-EGFR therapy.

The significance of HER2 in CRC therapeutic strategy is as follows:

(a) It serves as a biomarker of the resistance to anti-EGFR therapy and a negative predictive biomarker in CRC; (b) its overexpression/amplification shows poor response to anti-EGFR treatments; (c) it has a clear predictive role in determining EGFR inhibitor resistance; (d) it is more established as a negative predictive factor of anti-EGFR agent resistance [17, 30].

HER2 status can be assessed using immunohistochemistry (IHC) to determine protein expression as well as by in situ hybridization (ISH) to assess for HER2 gene amplification. HER2 overexpression is due to Erb-B2 amplification or the activation of somatic mutations and is defined in clinical practice as IHC3+ or IHC2+ and in situ hybridization (ISH)-positive disease. HER 2 overexpression is due to Errb2 amplification or the activation of somatic mutations [21].

6.3 CpG Island methylation phenotype (CIMP)

CIMP indicates hypermethylation in tumor suppressor/tumor-related genes and it can be classified as CIMP-High or CIMP-Low. The prognostic value of CIMP-positive tumor shows worse overall and disease-free survival with differential response to standard chemotherapeutic agents i.e., 5-FU and irinotecan [5]. Nevertheless, CIMP tumors frequently have concomitant mutations in BRAF or MSI, making CIMP involvement as an independent prognostic marker more challenging to interpret. It is difficult to interpret the contribution of CIMP as an independent prognostic marker [5].

Cancer with high DNA methylation can be categorized as CIMP positive, and it encompasses 35–40% of sporadic CRC cases. CpG hypermethylation can lead to silencing of tumor suppressor genes in carcinogenesis since the expression of the genes is repressed. In some cases, the presence of epigenetic silencing overlaps with MSI-H [6, 21, 31].

6.4 DNA methylation aberrations

Early changes in the pathogenesis of CRC can be identified through the presence of DNA methylation aberrations in cell-free DNA. For example, the sensitivity of hypermethylation of septin-9 (SEPT9) is 51–90% and the specificity is 73–96% in CRC patient's serum. However, SEPT9 sensitivity for advanced stage adenomas is merely 9.6%, limiting its functionality as a predictive biomarker [5]. Moreover, DNA aneuploidy, a surrogate marker of chromosomal instability, is associated with poor overall survival in stage II and III CRC as well as risk of early relapse in stage II CRC [5].

In addition, the loss of chromosome 18q associated with inactivation of tumor suppressor genes DCC, SMAD4, SMAD2, and CABLES1 results in low or poor overall survival of CRC. A meta-analysis highlighted survival in stage II CRC was 54% vs. 83% in the presence of 18q deletions.

In addition, over-expression of the pro-apoptotic *BCL-2* gene is associated with improved overall and disease-free survival in CRC, highlighting its potential as a prognostic marker [5].

6.5 Chromosome instability (CIN)

Most CRC arises through the CIN pathway due to loss/mutation of tumor suppressor genes and activation of oncogenes. The most commonly affected genes in CIN pathway are tumor suppressor genes such as adenomatous polyposis coli (APC) and p53, and oncogene KRAS, which all are responsible for the adenocarcinoma sequence pathway. Alterations within these genes can activate oncogenes mutation or deactivate tumor suppressors which will lead to malignant transformation. CIN pathway is proposed to be responsible for 80–85% of all CRC and adenomas [6].

6.5.1 Adenomatous polyposis coli gene (APC)

APC plays a significant role as the most important gatekeeper of colonic epithelial cell proliferation in the Wnt/Wingless pathway. It controls the underlying oncoprotein called B-catenin. The loss of APC gene function may trigger the transition from normal colonic mucosa to adenoma because of upregulation of B-catenin. Most sporadic colorectal adenomas and cancers have somatic APC mutations. They generally occur in 70% of sporadic CRCs and they are the roots of FAP cancer predisposition syndrome. WNT signaling is negatively regulated by APC protein through the facilitation of the targeting of the transcription factor B-catenin for ubiquitin-mediated proteasomal degradation. APC mutation in mCRC translates to poorer overall survival, which makes it useful to predict the clinical outcome of CRC [1]. And much like KRAS, APC mutation also appears in the early stages of the progression from adenoma to carcinoma [6, 31, 32].

6.5.2 TP53

TP53 is the most frequent somatic gene mutation, whose mutational status has been closely linked to positive response to adjuvant 5FU therapy in stage III CRC patients; although, further observations are required to determine TP53 role as a potential prognostic and predictive CRC biomarkers. Mutation in TP53 occurs in about half of all CRCs, and these mutations promote the malignant transformation of adenoma. Like APC, TP53 is a key tumor suppressor gene that has been extensively substantially studied in CRC, but it currently until now it still has no predictive or prognostic value role in the clinical setting. TP53 mutations or loss of function are reported in 50–75% of CRC cases [1, 21]. TP53 remains an important gene connected to with the progression adenoma-malignant tumor progression, and its loss of functions increase cell multiplication/proliferation and uncontrolled cell cycle (a pivotal step in the carcinogenesis of CRC) [22].

6.6 PIK3CA

PIK3CA is found in approximately 14–18% of CRC patients. It is one of the most frequently mutated oncogenes, but routine PIK3CA testing is not currently recommended for CRC patients. The existence of PTEN mutations, a tumor suppressor gene in PI3K/AKT/mTOR pathway, can result in increased metastatic risk and low survival rate [21]. Phosphatidylinositol-4,5-bisphosphate 3-kinase catalytic subunit alpha (*PIK3CA*) part of the PI3K/AKT/mTOR pathway has mutations in exon 9 or exon 20 in 10–15% cases [5].

6.7 Circulating free DNA (cfDNA)

CfDNA may be used to profile the molecular structure in early-stage of CRC patients, especially if tumor tissue is not available, although the clinical use of cfDNA in CRC patients is currently being investigated [17, 23]. FDA-approved screening test to detect cfDNA in the serum of CRC patients is based on Methylated Septin 9 (mSEPT9) DNA, as methylated biomarker. Detecting mSEPT9 in the plasma of CRC patients has been reported to be reliable to screen for CRC, it can also be found in precancerous lesions e.g., colorectal adenomas, but it may not have the reliable sensitivity [23].

The presence of circulating free DNA may indicate CRC, residual disease in CRC and other malignancies residuals. Therefore, cfDNA is associated with higher recurrence risk i.e. lower probability of recurrence-free and overall survival, and is useful in the planning of adjuvant treatment in metastatic CRC cases [5].

6.8 Consensus molecular subtypes (CMS)

Consensus molecular subtypes (CMS) categorize CRC into four molecular subtypes based on the biological differences in the profiles of the gene expression; and each of these four subtypes has different prognoses. CMS1 (MSI-like) group is marked by certain gene expression patterns such as d-MMR, MSI, and CIMP-high. CMS2 (canonical) includes CRC with activated Wnt and Myc signaling pathways. CMS3 (metabolic) groups CRC with metabolic dysregulation in various pathways with existing KRAS mutations and activated metabolic pathways. Finally, CMS4 (mesenchymal) CRC is characterized by a stromal invasion, angiogenesis, and upregulation of epithelial-mesenchymal transition genes [17, 21–23, 25].

6.9 Cancer stem cells (CSCs)

Contemporary chemotherapies generally target mature cancer cells. They can reduce the size of cancer tissue but cannot completely destroy cancer stem cells (CSCs) that have stronger self-renewing ability and resistance toward chemotherapy and radiotherapy compared to mature cancer cells. As such, when chemotherapy treatment is withdrawn, CR-CSCs that escape the therapy can grow into mature cancer cells, resulting in recurrence and metastasis [33].

Colorectal cancer stem cells (CR-CSCs) biomarkers can be valuable assets to develop CRC personalized treatment and tumor stratification by targeting the selected stem cell population. Mesenchymal stromal cells are known to have influential role on the therapy positive outcome, while resident stromal cells (RSCs) of tumor microenvironment (TME) appear to encourage the tumorigenic and metastatic processes [27].

CSCs are controlled by several pluripotent transcription factors such as OCT4, Sox2, Nanog, KLF4, and MYC. They are also regulated by different intracellular signaling pathways. These signaling pathways are: Wnt/β-catenin signaling pathways, NF-kB (nuclear factor-kB), Hedgehog (Hh), Notch, JAK/STAT (Janus kinase/signal transducers and activators of transcription), PI3K/AKT/mTOR (phosphoinositide 3-kinase/ AKT/ mammalian target of rapamycin), TGF (transforming growth factor)/ SMAD, and PPAR (peroxisome proliferator-activated receptor). Extracellular factors are also play a role, e.g., vascular niches, hypoxia, tumor associated macrophage (TAM), cancer-associated fibroblasts, cancer-associated mesenchymal stem cells, extracellular matrix, and exosomes [6, 26–28]. Several agents targeting CSCs and signaling pathways are being studied by many research facilities, such as: a) Napabucasin (targets the STAT3 pathway), b) Demcizumab (Anti-DLL4, inhibit the Notch pathway and CSC activity), c) Vismodegib (Hh pathway), d) R05429083 (CD44), e) AMC303 (CD44V6), etc. [6, 26–28].

Isolating the CR-CSCs is possible based on a group of CR-CSCs surface markers e.g., CD44, CD133, CD24, epithelial cell adhesion molecule (EpCAM), LGR5, and aldehyde dehydrogenase (ALDH). Since CR-CSCs are exceedingly tumorigenic, aggressive, radio-resistant and chemo-resistant, they play critical roles in CRC recurrence and metastasis. Thus, the development of new therapies targeting CR-CSCs by considering the tumor microenvironment (TME) and tumor metabolism may become an important research direction to overcome resistance to therapies [6, 26, 28, 34].

6.10 Tumor microenvironment (TME)

Tumor microenvironment (TME) includes various cell types such as cytotoxic and regulatory T-cells (CTL, Tregs), helper (Th) cells, natural killer (NK) cells, B-cells, myeloid-derived suppressor cells (MDSC), tumor-associated macrophages (TAM), cancer-associated fibroblasts (CAF), and endothelial cells. These cells provide anti- and pro-tumorigenic effects in their interaction with cancer cells, which play an important role in modulating tumor growth, invasion, and progression [1, 33].

CR-CSCs are located in a specific region of the TME known as CSC niche that preserves their properties and protects them from anti-cancer medications. TME and metabolic plasticity may be the culprit behind therapeutic failure by imposing selective pressures on CSCs [1, 26].

Recently, there has been mounting evidence that suggests the CRC microenvironment significantly supports or represses CRC progression and metastasis; hence, the importance of these non-cell-autonomous signaling pathways is more recognized [33].

TME alludes to a special biological environment constructed by malignant and non-malignant cells, and their discharged elements. It is mainly made up of cellular and non-cellular components that each have its own function but also work together during cancer progression and metastasis. The cellular components have cancerous and non-cancerous cells e.g., stromal myofibroblast, endothelial cells, immune cells (such as lymphocytes, macrophages, dendritic cells, neutrophils), and cancer-related fibroblast [26, 33]. The non-cellular component consists of the extracellular matrix (ECM), cytokine, growth factors and extracellular vesicles [26]. In the tumor stroma, cancer associated fibroblast secrete the cytokines CXCL1 and CXCL2 as well as interleukin-6, which promote angiogenesis and tumor progression [26]. In addition to these common components, intestinal cells are also in close contact with a large population of microorganisms referred to as the gut microbiota [33]. Published research found that there is a relationship between the expression levels of CD163 in Tumor Associated Macrophages (TAM) and the expression levels of colorectal cancer stem cell markers (CD133 and CD166) [35]. There is also previous research that studied CD133 expression and its correlation with clinicopathological profile of CRC patients in Medan, Indonesia. It reported that CD133 expressions were associated with the tumor location but not with other clinicopathological factors [36].

6.11 NTRK gene fusion panel

Neurotrophic tyrosine receptor kinase (NTRK) gene fusions are an actionable biomarker for cancer treatment. The presence of NTRK rearrangements in colorectal cancer patients is rare (<1%) but this actually might be used as a target to raise positive outcomes in NTRK-positive CRC patients.

To identify solid tumors while at the same time assessing any fusions occurring in the targeted regions of NTRK1, NTRK2, and NTRK 3 genes that result in fusion transcript, a comprehensive biomarker test such as The Next Gen Sequencing (NGS) can be utilized. The first-generation TRK inhibitors (Larotrectinib and entrectinib) have demonstrated efficacy and safety for mCRC patients showing signs of NTRK pathogenic fusions and having no alternative effective therapies.

NTRK-positive CRC patients is usually characterized by high tumor mutation burden, MSI-H, and poor prognosis [37, 38]. As previously stated, NTRK fusion is unusual; however, this information might be useful as a guidance for molecularly driven treatment, including targeted therapy and immunotherapy applicable to NTRK-positive CRC patients [39].

NTRK fusion screening test should also be recommended for patients with MSI-H or high TMB CRC [37]. CRC with NTRK fusions are described as having relation to APC and TP53 mutations, mutually exclusive with RAS/RAF alterations, frequently found in MSI-H/d-MMR CRCs [17]. mCRC with mutated NTRK commonly has wild-type RAS/BRAF and high MSI/d-MMR status; it is positively correlated with right-sidedness, female gender, old age, lymph node metastasis spread and worse prognosis. Larotrectnib and entrectinib are approved for the treatment of CRC exhibiting NTRK pathogenic fusions [39].

7. Conclusion

Biomarkers may serve as a therapeutic framework that influences the selection of the most suitable CRC treatment strategy. There are several biomarkers present in mCRC that can affect the success or failure of a chosen treatment, be it chemotherapy, targeted therapy or immunotherapy. These biomarkers include extended RAS (KRAS and NRAS), BRAFV600E mutation, d-MMR or microsatellite instability-high, and immune checkpoint or PD1, CTLA4, human EFGR2 (HER2) amplification, MEK, as well as actionable gene fusions such as neurotrophic tyrosine (tropomyosin) receptor kinase (NTRK) fusions/rearrangements.

NTRK is exceedingly rare but it may become the new target to better the outcomes of CRC treatment. The latest Next Generation Sequencing (NGS) method is able to discover all required genomic alteration types e.g., amplification, fusions, and MSI. MSI is a crucial biomarker for diagnostic, prognostic, and predictive purposes in CRC. The role of colorectal cancer stem cells (CR-CSCs) surface markers and target therapies to CR-CSCs and other types of biomarkers are currently being developed and continue to be researched by various researcher.

Author details

Rustam Effendi-YS[1*], Amido Rey[1] and Imelda Rey[2]

1 Columbia Asia Hospital, Medan, Indonesia

2 Faculty of Medicine, Department of Internal Medicine, Universitas Sumatera Utara, Medan, Indonesia

*Address all correspondence to: effendiysr@yahoo.com; rustamoreocr@gmail.com

References

[1] Effendi-YS R. Colonoscopy, biomarkers, and target therapy in colorectal cancer. Acta Medica Indonesiana – The Indonesian Journal of Internal Medicine. 2022;**54**(3):476-486

[2] Sung H, Ferlay J, Siegel RL, et al. Global cancer statistics 2020. Globocan estimates of incidence and mortality worldwide for 36 cancers in 185 countries. 04 February 2021. Cancer Journal for Clinicians. 2021;**71**(3):209-249

[3] Globocan. Indonesia-Global Cancer Observatory. 2020. Available from: https://gco.iarc.fr/today/factsheets/populations/360-indonesia-fact-sheets

[4] Effendi-YS R. Economic burden of colorectal cancer: Prevention vs treatment. In: Simadibrata M, Makmun D, Abdullah M, Syam AF, editors. Proceeding Book. Indonesian Digestive Disease Week (IDDW). Jakarta: Internal Publishing; 2016. pp. 50-58

[5] Ogunwobi O, Mahmood F, Akingboye A. Biomarkers in colorectal cancer; current research and future prospects. International Journal of Molecular Sciences. 2020;**21**(15):5311

[6] Effendi-YS R. Cancer stem cells and molecular biology tests in colorectal cancer: Therapeutic implications. Acta Medica Indonesiana – The Indonesian Journal of Internal Medicine. 2017;**49**(4):351-359

[7] Effendi-YS R. Adenomatous polyposis coli, mismatch repair, microsatellite instability in colorectal cancer based on locations [thesis]. Medan, Indonesia: Faculty of Medicine Universitas Sumatera Utara; 2013

[8] Effendi-YS R, Zain LH, Siregar G, et al. Adenomatous polyposis coli, mismatch repair, and microsatellite instability in colorectal cancer based on locations. Acta Medica Indonesiana – The Indonesian Journal of Internal Medicine. 2013;**45**(4):275-283. Available from: https://www.ncbi.nlm.nih.gov/pubmed/24448331#

[9] Shaukat A, Kahi CJ, Burk CA, Rabeneck L, Sauer BG, Rex DK. ACG clinical guidelines: Colorectal cancer screening 2021. The American Journal of Gastroenterology. 2021;**116**:458-479. DOI: 10.14309/ ajg.0000000000001122

[10] Crockett SD, Nagtegaal I. Terminology, molecular features, epidemiology, and management of serrated colorectal neoplasia. Gastroenterology. 2019;**157**(4):949-966.e4. DOI: 10.1053/j.gastro.2019.06.041. Epub 2019 Jul 16

[11] Effendi-YS R, Rey I. Molecular diagnosis in colorectal cancer. The Indonesian Journal of Gastroenterology, Hepatology, and Digestive Endoscopy. 2015;**16**(1):26-33

[12] Zamarin D, Saltz L. Colon cancer, rectal cancer. In: Drilon AE, Postow MA, Krug LM, editors. Pocket Oncol. Philadelpia: Wolters Kluwer. Lippincott William & Wilkins; 2014. pp. 156-159

[13] Effendi-YS R, Rey I, Khadafi M. Neoplasma usus besar (colorectal neoplasm). In: Effendi-YS R, editor. Penatalaksanaan Klinis Kelainan Gastrointestinal (Clinical Management of Gastrointestinal Disorders). Jakarta: EGC; 2019. pp. 263-276

[14] Hasler WL, Owyang C. Approach to the patient with gastrointestinal disease. In: Kasper DL, Fauci AS, Hauser SL, Longo DL, Jameson JL, Loscalzo JL,

editors. Harrison's Gastroenterology and Hepatology. 3rd ed. New York: McGraw-Hill Educ, Co. Inc.; 2017. pp. 80-88

[15] Nakayama G, Tanaka C, Kodera Y. Current options for the diagnosis, staging, and therapeutic management of colorectal cancer. Gastrointestinal Tumors. 2014;**I**:25-32. DOI: 10.1159/000354995

[16] Seal BS, Sullivan SD, Ramsey S, et al. Medical cost associated with use of systemic therapy in adults with colorectal cancer. Journal of Managed Care Pharmacy. 2013;**3**(2):65-75

[17] Puccini A, Seeber A, Berger MD. Biomarkers in metastatic colorectal cancer: Status quo and future perspective. Cancers. 2022;**14**(19):4828. DOI: 10.3390/cancers14194828

[18] Oh HN, Joo YH. Novel biomarkers for the diagnosis and prognosis of colorectal cancer. Intestinal Research. 2020;**18**(2):168-183

[19] Colorectal Cancer Biomarkers [2023 Patient Guide]. Available from: https://fightcolorectalcancer.org>

[20] Goel A. The era of biomarkers and preciccion medicine in colorectal cancer. Epigenomics. 2022;**14**(6):345-349. ISSN 1750-1911 34521. DOI: 10.2217/epi-2022-0010C2022

[21] Koncina E, Haan S, Rauh S, Letellier E. Prognostic and predictive molecular biomarkers for colorectal cancer: Updates and challenges. Cancer. 2020;**12**(2):319. DOI: 10.3390/cancers12020319

[22] Malki A, ElRuz RA, Gupta I, Allouch A, Vranic S, Al Moustafa AE. Molecular mechanisms of colon cancer progression and metastasis: Recent insights and advancements. International Journal of Molecular Sciences. 2021;**22**:130. DOI: 10.3390/ijms22010130

[23] Pang S-W, Awi NJ, Armon S, Lim WW-D, Low JS-H, Peh K-B, et al. Current update of laboratory molecular diagnostics advancement in management of colorectal cancer (CRC). Diagnostics. 2020;**10**:9. DOI: 10.3390/diagnostics10010009

[24] Piawah S, Venook AP. Targeted therapy for colorectal cancer metastases: A review of current methods of molecularly targeted therapy and the use of tumor biomarkers in the treatment of metastatic colorectal cancer. Cancer. 2019;**125**:4139-4147

[25] Xie YH, Chen YX, Fang JY. Comprehensive review of targeted therapy for colorectal cancer. Signal Transduction and Targeted Therapy. 2020;**5**:22. DOI: 10.1038/s41392-020-0116-z

[26] Hervieu C, Christou N, Battu S, et al. The role of cancer stem cells in colorectal cancer: From the basics to novel clinical trials. Cancers. 2021;**13**:1092. DOI: 10.3390/cancers13051092

[27] Patsalias A, Kozovska Z. Personalized medicine: Stem cells in colorectal cancer treatment. Biomedicine & Pharmacotherapy. 2021;**141**:111821. DOI: 10.1016/j.biopha.2021.11.111821

[28] Yang L, Shi P, Zhao G, et al. Targeting cancer stem cell pathway for cancer therapy. Signal Transduction and Targeted Therapy. 2020;**5**:8. DOI: 10.1038/s41392-020-0110-5

[29] Effendi-YS R, Rey I. Cancer stem cells and signaling pathways in colorectal cancer. Indonesian Journal of Gastroenterology, Hepatology, and Digestive Endoscopy. 2018;**19**(1):37-40

[30] Djaballah SA, Daniel F, Milani A, Ricagno G, Lonardi S. HER2 in colorectal cancer: The long and winding road from negative predictive factor to positive actionable target. American Society of Clinical Oncology Educational Book. Apr 2022;**42**(42). DOI: 10.1200/EDBK_351354

[31] Legolvan MP, Taliano RJ, Resnic MB. Application of molecular techniques in the diagnosis, prognosis and management of patients with colorectal cancer: A practical approach. Human Pathology. 2012;**43**:1157-1168

[32] Huth L, Jakel J, Dahl E. Molecular diagnostic applications in colorectal cancer. Microarrays. 2015;**3**:168-179

[33] Li J, Chen D, Shen M. Tumor microenvironment shapes colorectal cancer progression, metastasis, and treatment responses. Frontiers in Medicine. 2022;**9**:869010. DOI: 10.3389/fmed.2022.869010

[34] Ma YS, Li W, Liu Y, Shi Y, Lin QL, Fu D. Targeting colorectal cancer stem cells as an effective treatment for colorectal cancer. Technology in Cancer Research & Treatment. 2020;**19**:1-9. DOI: 10.1177/1533033819892261

[35] Rey I, Putra A, Lindarto D, Yusuf F. Relationship between CD163 tumor-associated macrophages and colorectal cancer stem cells markers. Open Access Macedonian Journal of Medical Sciences. Oct 2021;**9**(B):1381-1386. DOI: 10.3889/oamjms.2021.7188

[36] Rey I, Putra A, Yusuf F. Association between CD133 expression and clinicopathological profile in colorectal cancer. Medicinski Glasnik, May 2020;**17**(2):402-407. DOI: 10.17392/1106-20. Available from: https://www. Research gate.net/publication /341113802

[37] Wang H, Li ZW, Ou Q, Wu X, Nagasaka M, Shao Y, et al. NTRK fusion positive colorectal cancer is a unique subset of CRC with high TMB and microsatellite instability. Cancer Medicine. 2022;**11**(13):2541-2549. DOI: 10.1002/cam4.4561. Epub 2022 May 4

[38] Alese OB, Wu C, Chapin WJ, Ulanja MB, Zheng-Lin B, Amankwah M, et al. Update on emerging therapies for advanced colorectal cancer. American Society of Clinical Oncology Educational Book. 2023;**43**(43). DOI: 10.1200/EDBK_389574

[39] Ratti M, Grizzi G, Passalacqua LA, Cereatti F, Grassia R, et al. NTRK fusions in colorectal cancer: Clinical meaning and future perspective. Expert Opinion on Therapeutic Targets. 2021;**25**(8):677-683. DOI: 10.1080/14728222.2021.1978070

Chapter 3

Hypercholesterolemia Increases the Risk of Colorectal Cancer by a Tet-1-Dependent HSC-Autonomous Mechanism

Louis Messina and Guodong Tie

Abstract

The annual, age-standardized colorectal cancer (CRC) incidence rate has decreased by 46% from its peak in 1985. However, this long-standing decline in cases of CRC slowed due mainly to an increase in incidence in individuals younger than 50 years of age. For those less than 50 years of age, CRC is the leading cause of cancer deaths in men and the second in women. At least half of all cases of young-onset CRC are linked to lifestyle risk factors, including obesity. Hypercholesterolemia, a common metabolic disorder in obese people, has been shown to increase the risk of colorectal cancer, but the mechanism is unknown. We will show that hypercholesterolemia increases the incidence and pathological severity of colorectal cancer by inducing an oxidant stress-dependent hematopoietic stem cell-autonomous mechanism. The oxidized-LDL increase in HSC oxidant stress initiates a signaling pathway that culminates in the increased expression of miR101c that downregulates Tet1. This downregulation of Tet1 reduces the expression of the genes critical to the production and cytotoxicity of natural killer T cells and T cells, thereby impairing cancer immunosurveillance against colorectal cancer. This reveals a novel mechanism where a metabolic disorder induces epigenetic reprogramming of natural killer T cells and γδT gene expression within hematopoietic stem cells.

Keywords: colorectal cancer, hematopoietic stem cells, hypercholesterolemia, epigenetics, natural killer T cells and γδ T cells

1. Introduction

In 2024, colorectal cancer (CRC), the second most common cause of cancer death in the United States, is anticipated to cause 152,810 new cases of CRC and 53,010 deaths [1]. The annual, age-standardized CRC incidence rate has decreased by 46%, from 66.2 per 100,000 at its peak in 1985 to 35.7 per 100,000 persons in 2019. This decline is similar for men and women and occurred in large part due to the rapid dissemination of colonoscopy, reduced smoking, and more effective treatments [1].

However, this long-standing decline in cases of CRC has abated, driven largely by an increase in individuals younger than 55 years of age developing early-onset CRC at a more advanced stage and in the left colon/rectum [2]. For those less than 50 years of age, CRC is the leading cause of cancer death in men and the second leading cause of cancer death in women. Their presentation at a more advanced stage is attributed to the lack of screenings for that age group [1]. According to an analysis of the Surveillance, Epidemiology, and End Results (SEER) registry data, colon cancer incidence in Americans 20–34 years of age is anticipated to increase by 90% by 2030 and for rectosigmoid and rectal cancers by 124% [2].

The reasons for this devastating young onset of CRC have not yet been elucidated. Most do not have a genetic predisposition. For this reason, at least half of all cases of young-onset CRC are linked to lifestyle risk factors such as obesity, antibiotic use, and low physical activity. Diet may also be important in the development of young-onset CRC [3–5]. Identifying the pathogenetic mechanisms responsible for the young onset of CRC will permit the development of strategies to improve the clinical outcomes for this group of young patients.

Obesity will soon surpass smoking as the most preventable cause of cancer [6, 7]. Central or abdominal obesity doubles the risk of developing CRC [8]. The studies to determine which metabolic disorder in obese people is responsible for increasing their cancer risk have been unconvincing [9]. A common metabolic disorder in obese people, hypercholesterolemia, has been shown to increase cancer risk, including a significant increase in the risk of colorectal cancer [10]. Abdominal obesity and hypercholesterolemia synergically doubled the risk of CRC [8]. In addition, epidemiological investigations have found that the occurrence of CRC is positively correlated with a high-cholesterol diet [11, 12].

How hypercholesterolemia increases the risk of colorectal cancer has not been established. The mechanism linking hypercholesterolemia to CRC is usually attributed to its luminal effects by increased toxic bile acids and carcinogenic heterocyclic amines. Recently, a persuasive hypothesis has been advanced that hypercholesterolemia exerted a systemic and conditional influence that impaired the cellular components of tumor immunosurveillance [5, 8].

Hypercholesterolemia has also been shown to regulate the inflammatory response and innate immune response [13]. Additional support for the deleterious effects of hypercholesterolemia on the incidence of CRC comes from studies that show statin use can reduce the risk of overall colorectal cancer [14].

While hematopoietic stem cells maintain a quiescent undifferentiated state, they are subject to activating epigenetic enzymes and expression of lineage-associated genes, a process of lineage priming that maintains HSCs responsive to the physiologic and pathological demands for immune cell responses [15–18]. We have established that hypercholesterolemia profoundly affects HSC's most fundamental functions. We have shown that hypercholesterolemia induces oxidant stress in HSCs, accelerating their aging and impairing their repopulation capacity [19].

The primary effect of hypercholesterolemia on HSCs is to induce a receptor-mediated uptake of oxidized-low-density lipoprotein (ox-LDL) that increases the HSC oxidant stress that, in turn, activates the p38 MAPK pathway, which increases Notch1 [19]. This increased Notch expression induced a loss of quiescence, reducing the number of "long-term HSCs," undifferentiated pluripotent stem cells, and increased "short-term HSC," stem cells committed to various lineage specification pathways. In addition, hypercholesterolemia shortened telomeres and reduced their repopulation capacity. Together, these results show that hypercholesterolemia accelerates the aging of HSCs.

Based on these findings, we advanced the hypothesis that hypercholesterolemia induces an oxidized-LDL-dependent increase in HSC oxidant stress that reduces the production of innate immune cells that, in turn, impairs immunosurveillance against CRC.

2. The mechanisms by which hypercholesterolemia increases the incidence and pathological severity of colorectal neoplasia

2.1 Hypercholesterolemia increases the incidence and histopathologic severity of colorectal neoplasia by an HSC-autonomous mechanism

Colorectal neoplasia was induced with azoxymethane (AOM) in two mouse models of hypercholesterolemia, the ApoE−/− mouse and the C57BL/6 mouse fed a high cholesterol diet (HCD). The average tumor number was more than two-fold higher in hypercholesterolemic mice than in WT mice (**Figure 1A**). The histopathological stage of the tumors in hypercholesterolemic mice was also more advanced than in WT mice. The tumors in the hypercholesterolemic mice progressed to the late stages of tumorigenesis, including adenoma+++ and carcinoma stages. Meanwhile, the tumors at the early stages of tumorigenesis, including hyperplasia and adenoma+, were dramatically reduced in hypercholesterolemic mice (**Figure 1B**). Together, these results show that hypercholesterolemia increases the number and pathological severity of colorectal tumors [13].

To determine if hypercholesterolemia increases the incidence and pathologic severity of colorectal cancer by an HSC-autonomous mechanism, we transplanted HSCs from WT (CD45.2) and hypercholesterolemic mice into lethally irradiated WT mice (CD45.1). The serum cholesterol and white blood cell counts of the recipient WT mice were normal (**Figure 2D** and **E**). Remarkably, we found that the WT mice reconstituted with HSCs from hypercholesterolemic mice had nearly two-fold more tumors, and the histopathological severity was worse than that in WT mice reconstituted with WT HSCs (**Figure 1C** and **D**). These results show that hypercholesterolemia increases the incidence and pathologic severity of colorectal tumors by an HSC-autonomous mechanism.

2.2 Hypercholesterolemia specifically reduces the differentiation of HSCs toward NKT and γδ T cells

Given that hypercholesterolemia increases the incidence of colorectal neoplasia by an HSC-autonomous mechanism, we hypothesized that hypercholesterolemia impairs HSC production of immune cells that weakens cancer immunosurveillance against colorectal neoplasia. We found that NKT and γδ T cells were significantly reduced in number in the circulation. While these cells are rare in circulation and secondary lymphoid tissue, they are enriched in many peripheral tissues, such as the skin, intestines, and lungs. They are critical in the colon submucosa's response to infection and tumors. NKT and γδ T cells are unique because they exhibit innate and adaptive immune responses. NKT and γδ T cells secrete various cytokines critical for the antitumor functions of cytotoxic T cells. NKT and γδ T cells also interact with antigen-presenting cells to induce them to secrete cytokines that recruit and stimulate the antitumor functions of cytotoxic T cells, boosting innate and adaptive antitumor responses [19–21].

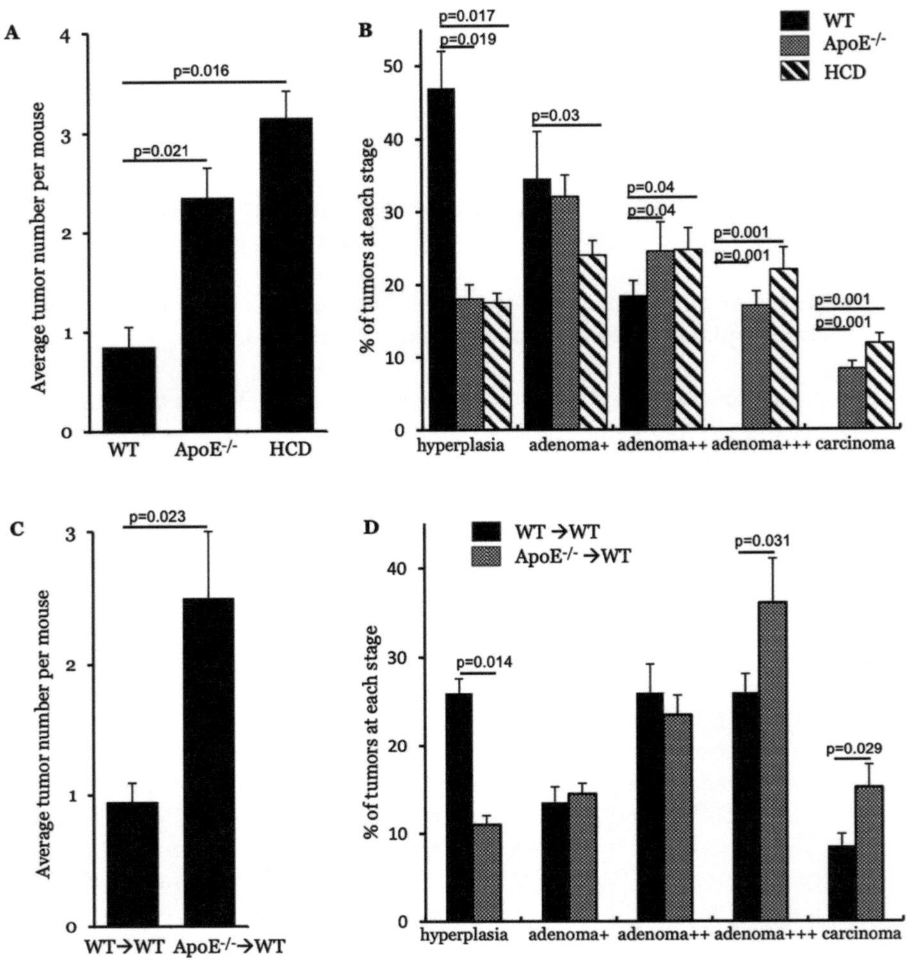

Figure 1.
*Hypercholesterolemia increases the average tumor number and histopathologic stage of colorectal neoplasia through a hematopoietic stem cell-autonomous manner. A. Average tumor number per mouse from WT, ApoE-/-, and HCD mice. B. Histopathologic stages of the tumors from WT, ApoE-/-, and HCD mice. n=12, *, p<0.05; **, p<0.01, vs. WT. C. Average tumor number from WT recipient mice reconstituted with HSCs from WT or ApoE-/- mice. D. Histopathologic stages of the tumors from WT recipient mice reconstituted with HSCs from WT or ApoE-/- mice. n=12, *, p<0.05; **, p<0.01, vs. WT [13].*

NKT and γδ T cell concentrations were also reduced in the thymus of hypercholesterolemic mice (**Figure 3A** and **B**). At phases 1 $CD44^-NK1.1^-$] and 2 [$CD44^+NK1.1^-$; intrathymic NKT-cell development in hypercholesterolemic mice was identical to WT (**Figure 4C**) as was the CD4+ subsets of NKT cells (**Figure 4D**). In all of the mouse models, the T-cell developmental intermediates were similar (**Figure 4E** and **F**) FACS analysis did not show any significant change in CDe3+, CD4+, and CD8+ T-cell populations in the peripheral blood of hypercholesterolemic mice apart from a slight decrease in B cells and a slight increase in NK cells (**Figure 4G**). In lethally irradiated WT recipient mice that were reconstituted with HSCs from hypercholesterolemic mice, we observed in the thymus an almost identical decrease in the HSC differentiation toward γδ T cells and NKT cells as that seen in hypercholesterolemic mice (**Figure 3C** and **D**). Thus, hypercholesterolemia induces an HSC-autonomous reduction in the production of HSCs toward NKT and γδ T cells [13].

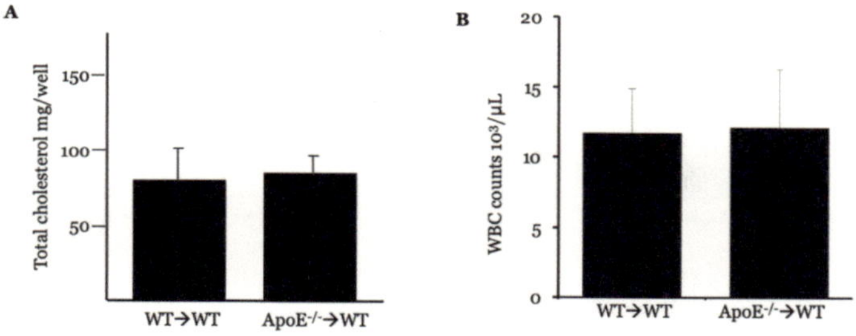

Figure 2.
WT recipient mice reconstituted with HSCs from hypercholesterolemic ApoE-/- mice have normal serum cholesterol levels and white blood cell counts. A. Serum cholesterol levels of WT recipient mice reconstituted with HSCs from WT or ApoE-/- mice. B. White blood cell counts of WT recipient mice reconstituted with HSCs from WT or ApoE-/- mice [13].

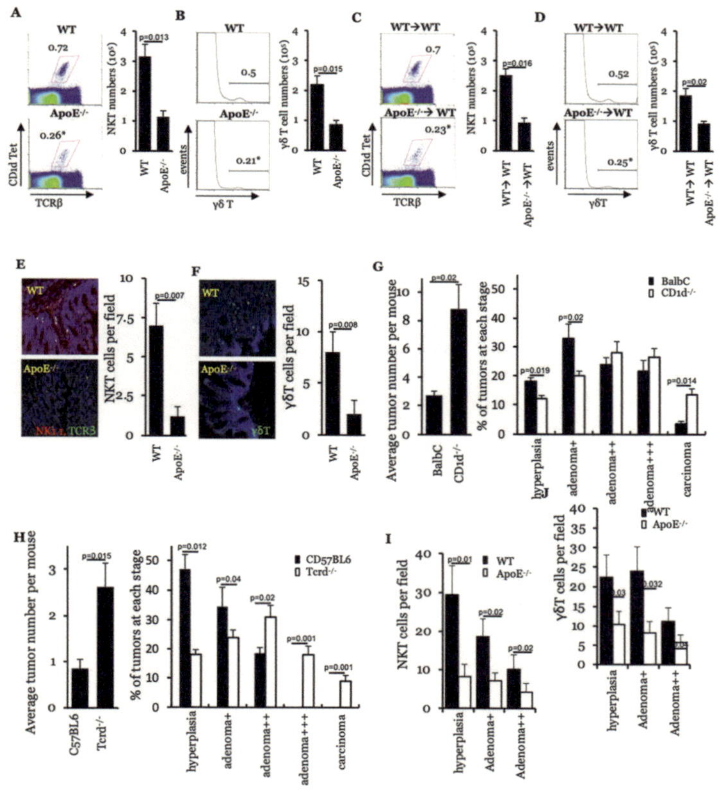

Figure 3.
Hypercholesterolemia significantly impairs the differentiation of HSCs towards NKT and γδT cells which are critical components of innate immunity against colorectal neoplasia. A. Hypercholesterolemia significantly impairs the differentiation of HSCs toward NKT and γδT cells, which are critical components of innate immunity against colorectal neoplasia. A, Frequency and total number of NKT cells in thymus of WT and ApoE-/- mice. n = 8. B. Frequency and total number of γδT cells in thymus of WT and ApoE-/- mice. n = 8. C. Frequency and total number of NKT cells in thymus of lethally irradiated WT recipients reconstituted with HSCs from WT or ApoE-/- mice. n = 8. D. Frequency and total number of γδT cells in thymus of lethally irradiated WT recipients reconstituted with HSCs from WT or ApoE-/- mice. n = 8. E. Frequency of submucosal NKT cells in colon of WT and ApoE-/- mice. n = 8. F. Frequency of submucosal γδT cells in colon of WT and ApoE-/- mice. n = 8. G. Average tumor number and histopathologic stage of AOM-induced colorectal neoplasia in CD1d-/- mice. n = 10. H. Average tumor number and histopathologic stages of AOM-induced colorectal neoplasia in Tcrd-/- mice. n = 10. I. Frequency of NKT cells in the tumors from WT and ApoE-/- mice. n = 8. J, Frequency of γδT cells in the tumors from WT and ApoE-/- mice. n = 8 [13].

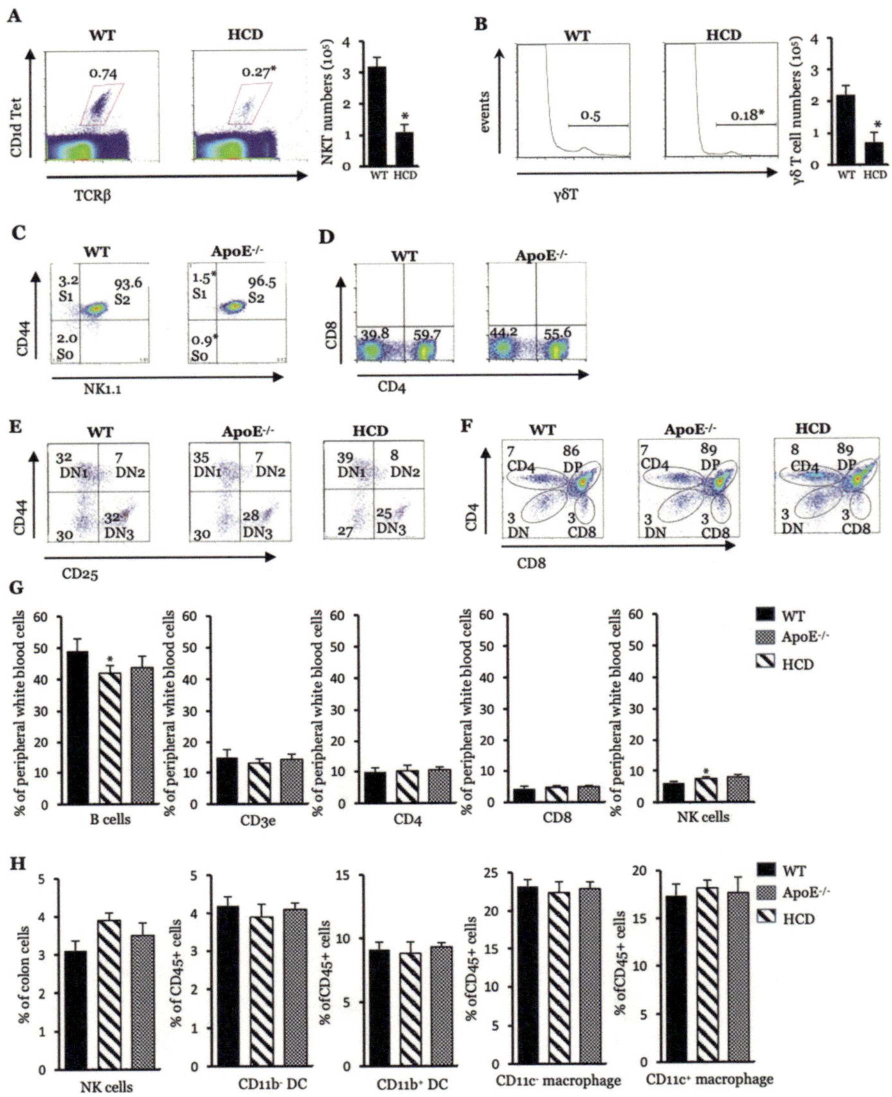

Figure 4.

*Hypercholesterolemia reduces the frequency and alters specific subsets and maturation of NKT and γδT cells in the thymus. A. Frequency and number of NKT cells in thymus of WT and HCD mice. n=6, *, p<0.05, vs. WT. B. Frequency and number of γδT cells in thymus of WT and HCD mice. n=6, *, p<0.05, vs. WT. C. DN1 (CD44+CD25–DN), DN2 (CD44+CD25+DN) and DN3 (CD44–CD25+DN) populations in thymus of WT, ApoE-/- and HCD mice. n=8, *, p<0.05, vs. WT. D. DP (CD4+CD8+), DN (CD4-CD8-), CD4+ and CD8+ populations in thymus of WT, ApoE-/- and HCD mice. n=8, *, p<0.05, vs. WT. E. Stage 0 (CD44-NK1.1-), Stage 1 (CD44+NK1.1-) and Stage 2 (CD44+NK1.1+) of NKT cells in thymus of WT and ApoE-/- mice. F, CD4+ and CD4-CD8- subsets of NKT cells in thymus of WT and ApoE-/- mice. n = 5, *, p<0.05, vs. WT. G. Frequency of B cells, NK cells, CD3e+, CD4+ and CD8+ cells in peripheral blood of WT, ApoE-/- and HCD mice. n = 5, *, p<0.05, vs. WT. H. NK cells (CD45+CD3e-NKp46+), CD11b- dendritic cells (CD11c+CD11b-CD103+F4/80-), CD11b+ dendritic cells (CD11c+CD11b+CD103+F4/80-), CD11c- macrophages (CD11c-CD11b+CD103-F4/80+) and CD11c+ macrophages (CD11c+CD11b+CD103-F4/80+) in the colon of WT, ApoE-/- and HCD mice. n = 5, *, p<0.05, vs. WT [13].*

In harmony with these findings in the thymus, in the colon submucosa of hypercholesterolemic mice, we found a substantial reduction of NKT cells [up to 6-fold] and γδ T cells [3-fold] (**Figure 3E** and **F**). In the meantime, we found in the colon of hypercholesterolemic mice that the other major cellular components of cancer immunosurveillance, including NK cells, CD11b⁻ dendritic cells, CD11b⁺ dendritic cells, CD11c⁻ macrophages, and CD11c⁺ macrophages did not show any meaningful changes (**Figure 4H**).

2.3 NKT and γδ T cells are critical components of immunosurveillance against colorectal neoplasia induced by azoxymethane

To provide additional support for our hypothesis that NKT and γδ T cells play a critical role in immunosurveillance against colorectal neoplasia, colorectal neoplasia was induced with azoxymethane in mice which lack γδ T cells (Tcrd−/− mice), and in mice which lack NKT cells (CD1d−/−mice). Both mouse strains showed a much higher incidence and greater histopathologic severity of colorectal neoplasia than that documented in their control background strains (**Figure 3G** and **H**). We also showed significantly lower concentrations of NKT and γδ T cells in the early but not later stages of tumorigenesis in hypercholesterolemic mice than that in WT mice (**Figure 3I** and **J**). These findings show that hypercholesterolemia reduced the concentrations of NKT and γδ T cells, which impaired tumor immunosurveillance against colorectal neoplasia [13].

2.4 The incidence of colorectal neoplasia is a linear function of hypercholesterolemia-induced HSC oxidant stress

Hypercholesterolemia induced a receptor-mediated uptake of oxidized-LDL that induced HSC oxidant stress that profoundly affected normal HSC function, accelerating their aging and reducing their repopulation capacity [19]. These effects were reduced by the administration of N-acetylcysteine [NAC]. Therefore, we hypothesized that NAC would also reverse the effects of hypercholesterolemia on NKT and γδ T cell number and cancer immunosurveillance. In pursuit of this possibility, we confirmed in hypercholesterolemic mice that NAC also rescued the impaired differentiation of HSCs toward NKT and γδ T cells (**Figure 5A** and **B**). In addition, NAC significantly decreased the average tumor number in both ApoE−/− and HCD mice. While NAC reduced the histopathologic severity of tumors in HCD mice, the reduction in the histopathologic severity of tumors in ApoE−/− mice did not reach statistical significance (**Figure 5C** and **D**). In both ApoE−/− and HCD mice, NAC also increased the infiltration of NKT and γδ T cells in the early stages of tumorigenesis (**Figure 5E** and **F**). Linear regression analysis between the level of HSC oxidant stress and the number of tumors per mouse revealed an incredible linear correlation between these variables [$r^2 = 0.87$] (**Figure 5G**). These findings reveal that hypercholesterolemia-induced hematopoietic stem cell oxidant stress directly mediates the reduction of HSC production of NKT and γδ T cells, and this reduction in NKT and γδ T cells in tumor number and their histopathological severity [13].

2.5 Hypercholesterolemia-induced downregulation of Tet1 in HSCs impairs their differentiation toward NKT and γδ T cells

Since the effects of hypercholesterolemia on NKT and γδ T cells are cell-autonomous and sustained after transplantation into WT mice who have normal cholesterol levels, there are at least two possible molecular mechanisms: oxidative stress-induced DNA mutations or oxidative stress-induced changes in epigenetic enzyme expression.

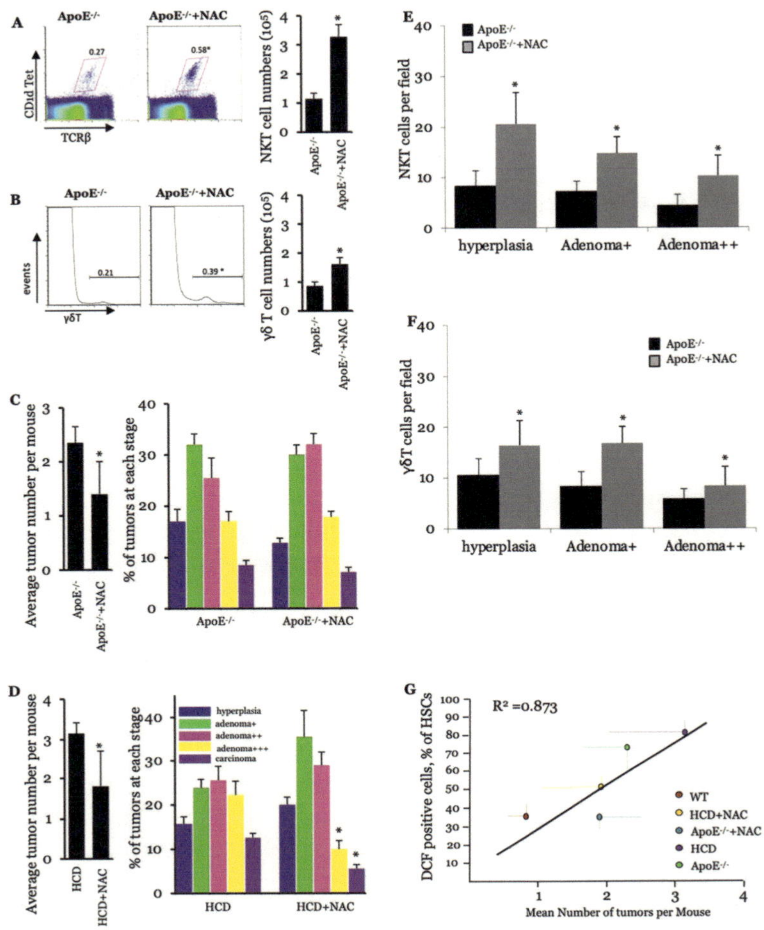

Figure 5.
*Hypercholesterolemia-induced oxidant stress in HSCs strongly correlates with the incidence of AOM-induced colorectal neoplasia. A. Frequency and total number of NKT cells in thymus of ApoE-/- and N-Acetyl Cysteine (NAC) treated ApoE-/- mice. n=8, *, p<0.05, vs. ApoE-/-. NAC was given in drinking water for 8 weeks (150mg/kg/day). B. Frequency and total number of γδT cells in thymus of ApoE-/- and NAC treated ApoE-/- mice. n=8, *, p<0.05, vs. ApoE-/-. C. Average tumor number and histopathologic stages of tumors isolated from ApoE-/- and NAC treated ApoE-/- mice. n=12, *, p<0.05, vs. ApoE-/-. D. Average tumor number and histopathologic stages of tumors isolated from High Cholesterol Diet (HCD) and NAC treated HCD mice. n=12, *, p<0.05, vs. HCD. E. NKT cell infiltration in the early stages of tumorigenesis in ApoE-/- and NAC treated ApoE-/- mice. n=6, *, p<0.05, vs. ApoE-/- . F. γδ T cell infiltration in the early stages of tumorigenesis in ApoE-/- and NAC treated ApoE-/- mice. n=12, *, p<0.05, vs. ApoE-/-. G. Regression analysis between oxidant stress in HSCs and tumor number [13].*

We found oxidant stress-dependent reduction in the expression of Tet1 in HSCs from hypercholesterolemic mice (**Figure 6A** and **B**). Tet2 has been shown to regulate key HSC functions, including self-renewal, proliferation, and hematopoiesis [22–24]. However, the role of tet1 in these key HSC functions is unknown. In order to determine if Tet1 plays a direct role in the reduced production of NKT and γδ T cells and the consequent impairment of tumor immunosurveillance, we determined the proportion and number of NKT and γδ T cells in the thymus of WT and Tet1−/− mice. As we found in hypercholesterolemic mice, the proportion and number of NKT and γδ T cells in the thymus of Tet1−/− mice was significantly lower than that of WT mice

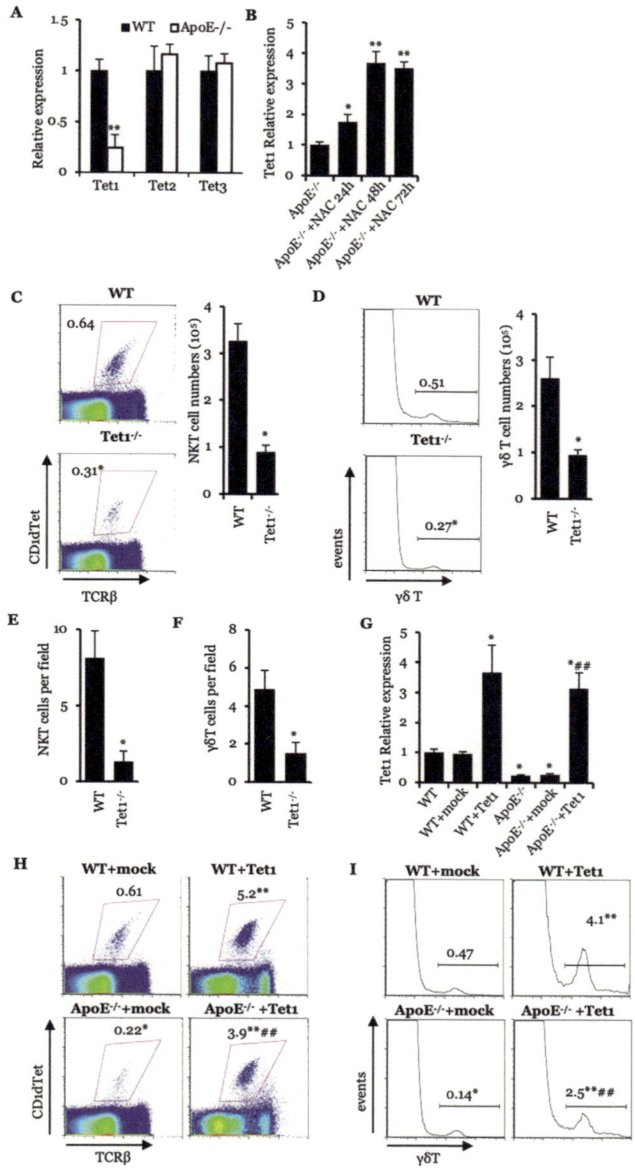

Figure 6.

*Hypercholesterolemia-induced oxidant stress in HSCs positively correlates with AOM-induced colorectal neoplasia. A. Expression of Tet1, Tet2, and Tet3 in HSCs from WT and ApoE-/- mice; n = 6, **, P < 0.01, versus WT. B. Downregulation of Tet1 expression in HSCs from ApoE-/- is oxidant stress dependent in mice; n = 6, *P < 0.05; **, P < 0.01, versus ApoE-/-. C. Frequency and number of NKT cells in thymus of WT and Tet1-/- mice; n = 5. *, P < 0.05, versus WT. D. Frequency and number of γδT cells in thymus of WT and Tet1-/- mice; n = 5. *, P < 0.05, versus WT. E. Frequency of submucosal NKT cells in colon of WT and Tet1-/- mice; n = 5, *, P < 0.05, versus WT. F. Frequency of submucosal γδT cells in colon of WT and Tet1-/- mice. n = 5; *, P < 0.05, versus WT. G. Tet1-relative expression following its overexpression in WT and Apoe-/- HSCs. n = 6; *, P < 0.05, versus WT; ##, P < 0.01, versus ApoE-/-. H. Frequency of NKT cells in thymus of recipient mice transplanted with WT HSCs, ApoE-/- HSCs, Tet1-overexpressing WT HSCs, or Tet1-overexpressing ApoE-/- HSCs. n = 6; *, P < 0.05; **, P < 0.01, versus WT+Mock; ##, P < 0.01, versus ApoE-/-+Mock. I. Frequency of γδT cells in thymus of recipient mice transplanted with WT HSCs, ApoE-/- HSCs, Tet1-overexpressing WT HSCs, or Tet1-overexpressing ApoE-/- HSCs. n = 6; *, P < 0.05; **, P < 0.01, versus WT+Mock; ##, P < 0.01, versus ApoE-/-+Mock [13].*

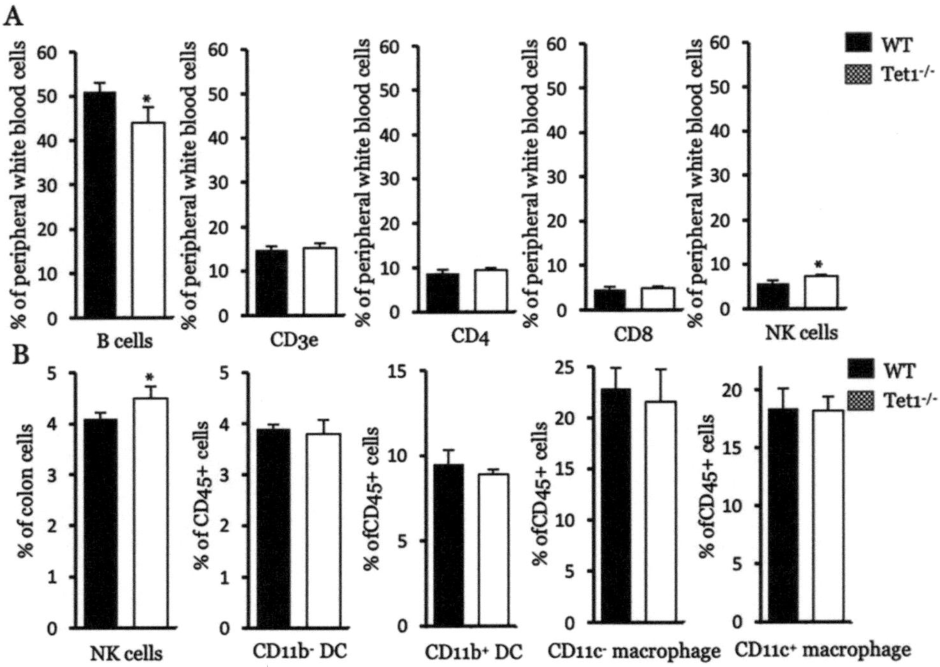

Figure 7.
*Frequency of T cell intermediate populations in thymus and cellular components responsible for cancer immunosurveillance in peripheral blood and colon of WT and Tet-/- mice. A. Frequency of B cells, NK cells, CD3e+, CD4+ and CD8+ cells in peripheral blood of WT and Tet1-/- mice. n = 6, *, p<0.05, vs. WT. B. NK cells (CD45+CD3e-NKp46+), CD11b- dendritic cells (CD11c+CD11b-CD103+F4/80-), CD11b+ dendritic cells (CD11c+CD11b+CD103+F4/80-), CD11c- macrophages (CD11c-CD11b+CD103-F4/80+) and CD11c+ macrophages (CD11c+CD11b+CD103-F4/80+) in the colon of WT and Tet1-/- mice. n = 6, *, p<0.05, vs. WT [13].*

(**Figure 6C** and **D**). Also consistent with our findings in hypercholesterolemic mice, the proportion and number of NKT and γδ T cells in the colon submucosa of Tet1−/− mice was substantially lower than that in WT mice (**Figure 6E** and **F**). We did not find any changes in the peripheral blood of Tet1−/− mice CD3e+. CD4+, or CD8+ cells. We found a slight decrease in B cells and NK cells in Tet1−/− mice (**Figure 7A** and **B**).

In contrast to these findings to these findings in Tet1 knockout mice, we found that overexpression of Tet1in HSCs from WT and hypercholesterolemic mice resulted in a 7-fold increase of NKT cells in WT mice and an almost 20-fold increase in NKT cells hypercholesterolemic mice, in vivo and in vitro. In parallel finding, overexpression of Tet1in HSCs from WT and hypercholesterolemic mice resulted in a 10-fold increase in WT and a 20-fold increase in γδ T cells (**Figures 6G–I** and **8A, D** and **E**). These results support the novel and specific role of Tet1 in HSCs lineage specification toward NKT and γδ T cells.

Given these effects of overexpression of Tet1 on the production of γδ T cells we sought to test the hypothesis that overexpression of Tet1 in hypercholesterolemic mice would restore the production of NKT and γδ T cells and thereby immunosurveillance against colorectal neoplasia. To this end, we reconstituted lethally irradiated WT mice with HSCs from WT and ApoE−/− mice that overexpress Tet1. Unexpectedly, lethally irradiated mice reconstituted HSCs that overexpressed Tet1,

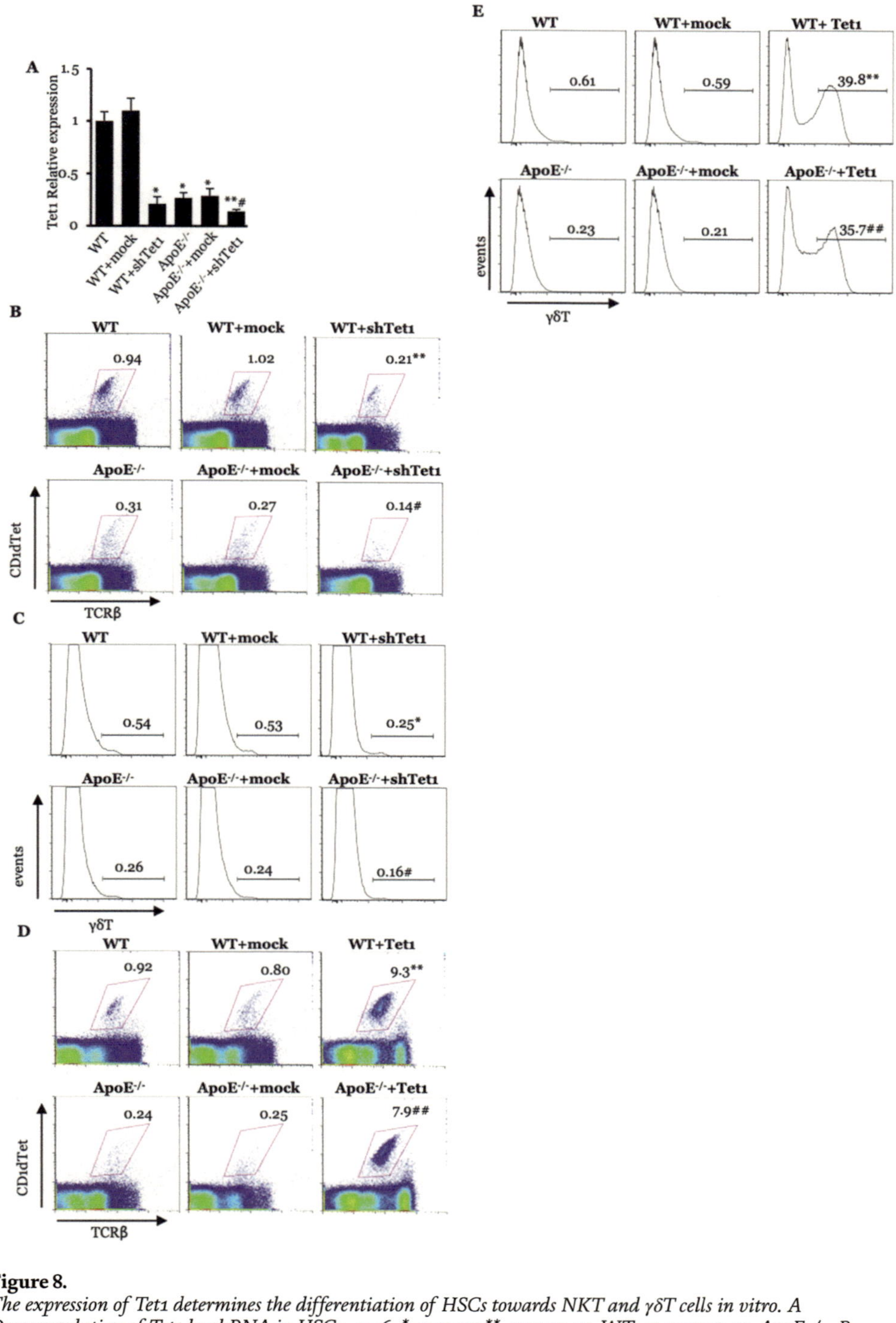

Figure 8.
*The expression of Tet1 determines the differentiation of HSCs towards NKT and γδT cells in vitro. A Downregulation of Tet1 by shRNA in HSCs . n=6, *, p<0.05; **, p<0.01, vs. WT; #, p<0.05, vs. ApoE-/-. B Differentiation of HSCs towards NKT cells in vitro following Tet1 downregulation C. Differentiation of HSCs towards γδT cells in vitro following Tet1 downregulation. n=6, *, p<0.05; **, p<0.01, vs. WT; #, p<0.05, vs. ApoE-/-. D. Differentiation of HSCs towards NKT cells in vitro following Tet1 overexpression E. Differentiation of HSCs towards γδT cells in vitro following Tet1 overexpression. n=6, *, p<0.05; **, p<0.01, vs. WT; #, p<0.05, vs. ApoE-/- [13].*

and all died. To address this problem, we included 1/3 non-transduced HSCs. Under these conditions, all mice survived, indicating clearly that Tet1 has an important role in HSC engraftment after irradiation. Overexpression of Tet1 in the HSCs of hypercholesterolemic mice restored the concentration of NKT and γδ T cells in the thymus and colon submucosa to that in WT mice (**Figure 9A–E**). Perhaps our most important finding is, overexpression of Tet1 in HSCs from hypercholesterolemic mice reduced the number of colorectal tumors by 55%, similar to that in WT mice (**Figure 9F–G**). Overexpression of Tet1 in HSCs of hypercholesterolemic also greatly reduced the histopathological severity of the colorectal neoplasia (**Figure 9G**). In WT and hypercholesterolemic mice, overexpression of Tet1 eliminated the progression of tumors to the carcinoma stage.

These results show that the mechanism by which hypercholesterolemia increases the risk of colorectal neoplasia is by inducing a Tet1-dependent HSC-autonomous mechanism that epigenetically reprograms the number and gene expression of NKT and γδ T cells. Given the unexpected simplicity of this finding, it could be leveraged into the creation of a cell immunotherapy for a variety of cancers.

2.6 MiR101c mediates the downregulation of Tet1 in HSCs isolated from hypercholesterolemic mice

We have shown that hypercholesterolemia induces an oxidized-LDL-dependent increase in HSC oxidant stress that initiates a signaling pathway culminating in the reduction to Tet1. How is Tet1 directly regulated? To address this question, we performed miRNA microarray analysis in HSCs isolated from WT and ApoE−/− mice (**Figure 10A**). MiR101c, predicted to target Tet1 directly, was upregulated significantly in HSCs from ApoE−/− mice. This increased level of miR101c was validated by RT-PCR (**Figures 10B** and **11A**). Application of NAC effectively reduced the overexpression of miR101c in HSCs from ApoE−/− mice (**Figures 10B** and **11A**). Overexpression of miR101c in HSCs from WT and hypercholesterolemic mice greatly reduced Tet1 expression (**Figure 11B** and **C**). Transfection of an inhibitor of miR101c greatly increased Tet1 expression (**Figure 11D** and **E**). In a luciferase assay of the Tet1 3′-UTR, miR101c reduced luciferase activity, whereas when the Tet1 binding sites were blocked, miR101c failed to increase luciferase activity (**Figure 11F**) These findings indicate that miR101c directly binds to the 3′-UTR of Tet1.

2.7 Tet1 directly induces the expression of genes critical for HSC differentiation toward NKT and γδ T cells

While the detailed mechanism by which HSCs produce NKT and γδ T cells remains incompletely described, a group of genes has been shown to be critical to this process [25, 26]. We sought to characterize the effects of Tet1 on the expression and epigenetic regulation of these genes that are required for HSC production of NKT and γδ T cells (**Table 1**). Of these genes, five, Fyn, Sox13, IL15R, ITK, and SH2D1a, had lower expression in ApoE−/− HSCs than in WT HSCs (**Figure 12A**). When Tet1 was overexpressed in HSCs from WT and ApoE−/− mice, their expression increased substantially (**Figure 12A**). Because Tet1 regulates the methylation of genes [23, 27], we proceeded to use pyrosequencing to characterize the effects of Tet1 on the methylation at key regulatory regions of these five genes that were affected

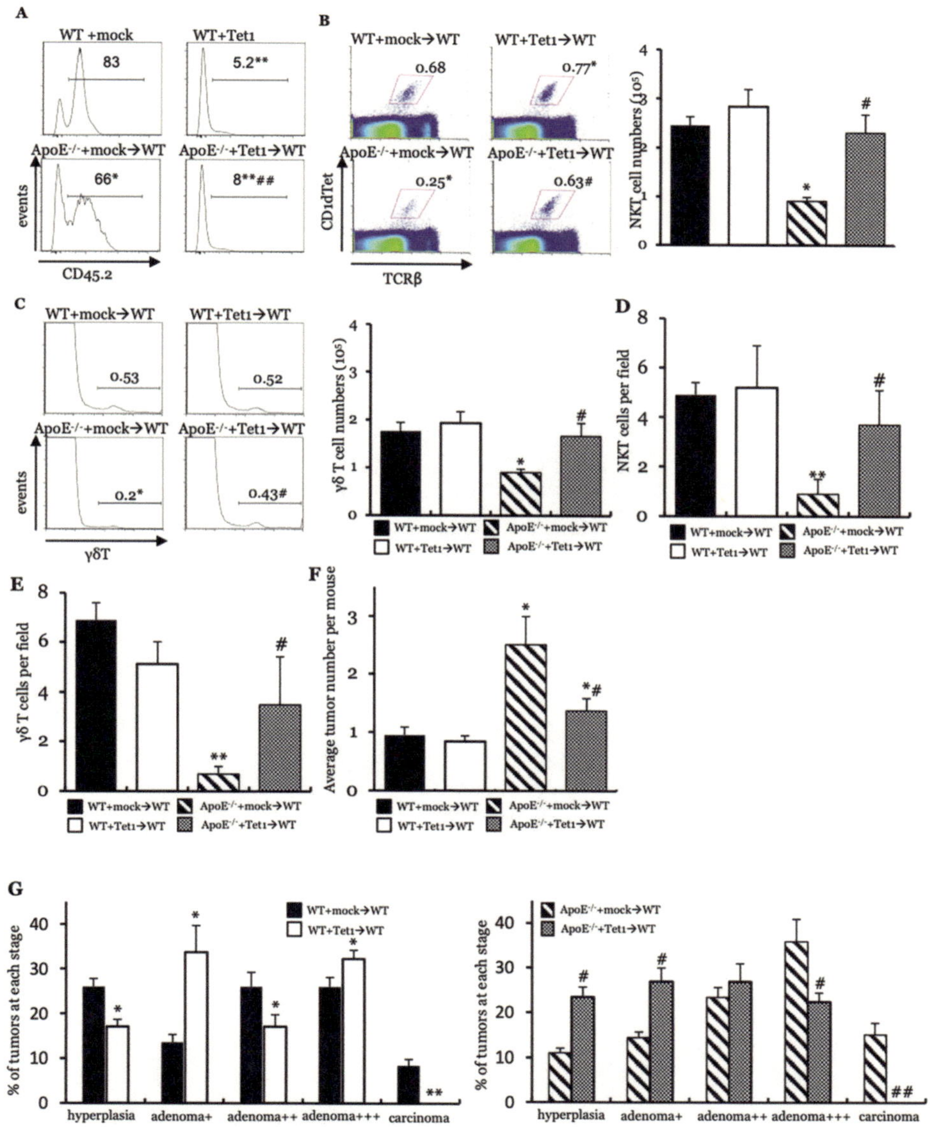

Figure 9.
*Hypercholesterolemia induced oxidant stress downregulates the expression of Tet1 in HSCs that impairs their differentiation towards NKT and γδT cells. A. Frequency of cells derived from Tet1-overexpressing HSCs. The transplantation of Tet1-overexpressing WT HSCs was supported with WT HSCs and the transplantation of Tet1-overexpressing ApoE-/- HSCs was supported with ApoE-/- HSCs, both at the ratio of 3:1. n = 8; *, P < 0.05; **, P < 0.01, versus WT+Mock; ##, P < 0.01, versus ApoE-/-+Mock. B. Frequency and total number of NKT cells in thymus of the recipients after transplantation with WT HSCs, ApoE-/- HSCs, Tet1-overexpressing WT HSCs+WT HSCs, or Tet1-overexpressing ApoE-/- HSCs+ApoE-/- HSCs. n = 8; *, P < 0.05, versus WT+Mock→WT; #, P < 0.05, versus ApoE-/-+Mock→WT. C. Frequency and total number of γδT cells in thymus of the recipients. n = 8; *, P < 0.05, versus WT+Mock→WT; #, P < 0.05, versus ApoE-/-+Mock→WT. D. Frequency of NKT cells in colon submucosa of the recipients. n = 8; **, P < 0.01, versus WT+Mock→WT; #, P < 0.05, versus ApoE-/-+Mock→WT. E. Frequency of γδT cells in colon submucosa of the recipients. n = 8; **, P < 0.01, versus WT+Mock→WT; #, P < 0.05, versus ApoE-/-+Mock→WT. F. Average tumor number per mouse in the recipients. n = 12; *, P < 0.05, versus WT+Mock→WT; #, P < 0.05, versus ApoE-/-+Mock→WT. G. Histopathologic stages of tumors. n = 12; *, P < 0.05; **, P < 0.01 versus WT+Mock→WT; #, P < 0.05; ##, P < 0.01, versus ApoE-/-+Mock→WT [13].*

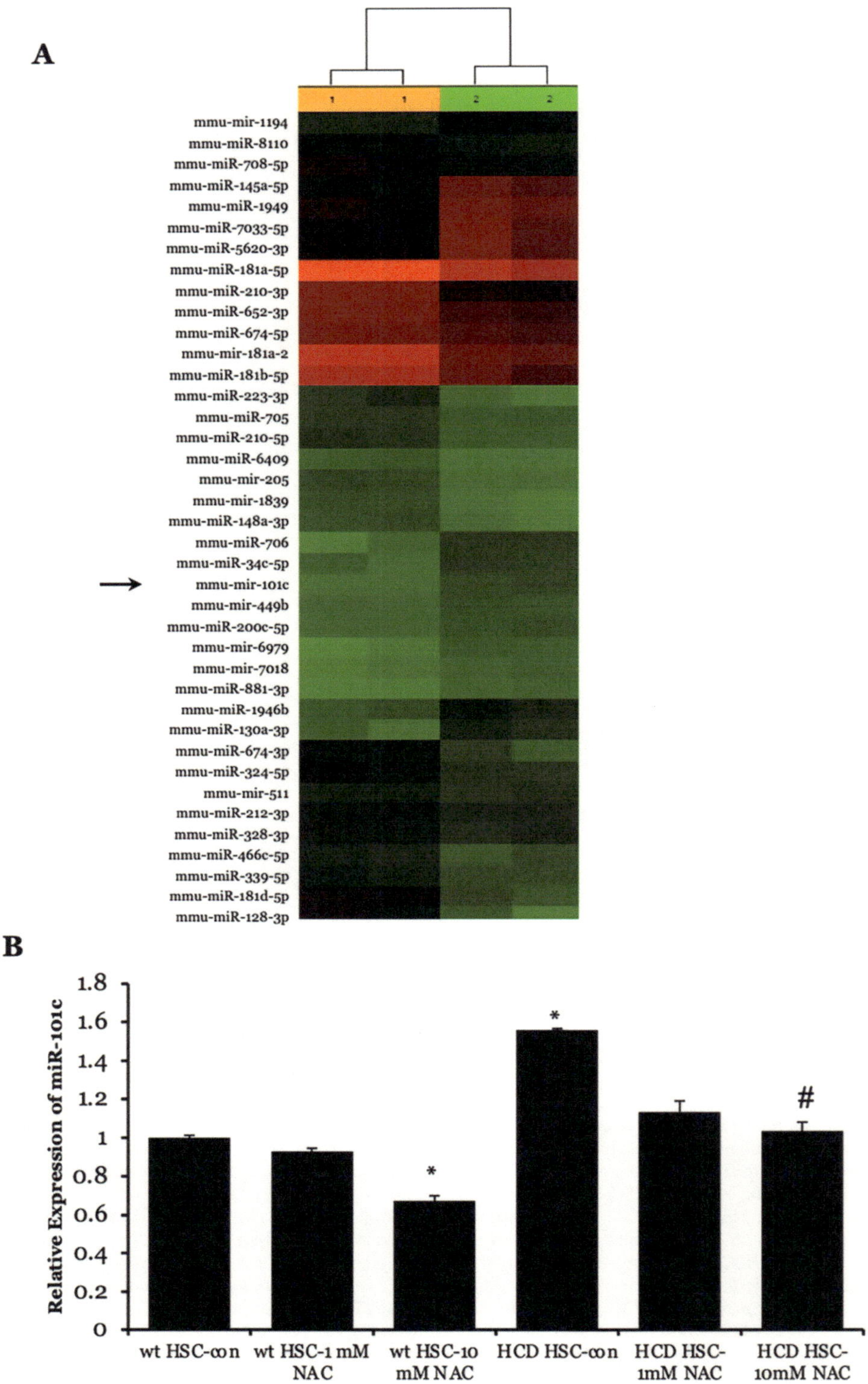

Figure 10.

*Expression of miRNA in HSCs from hypercholesterolemic mice. A. Microarray profiling analysis in HSCs from WT and ApoE-/- mice. n=4. B. Oxidant stress dependent upregulation of miR-101c expression in HSCs from HCD fed mice. n=4, *, p<0.05, vs WT control; #, p<0.05, vs HCD control [13].*

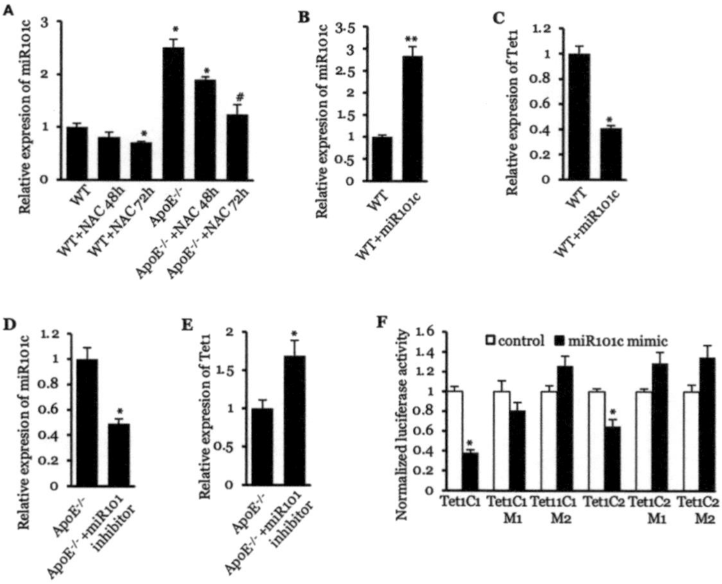

Figure 11.
*Reconstitution of lethally irradiated WT mice with ApoE-/- HSCs that overexpress Tet1 restores immunosurveillance against colorectal neoplasia. A. The frequency and total number of NKT cells in thymus and blood of the recipients after transplantation with WT HSCs, ApoE-/- HSCs, Tet1-overexpressing WT HSCs+ WT HSCs, or Tet1-overexpressing ApoE-/- HSCs+ApoE-/- HSCs. n=8, *, $p<0.05$, vs. WT→WT; #, $p<0.05$, vs. ApoE-/-→WT. B. The frequency and total number of $\gamma\delta$T cells in thymus and blood of the recipients. n=8, *, $p<0.05$, vs. WT→WT; #, $p<0.05$, vs. ApoE-/-→WT. C. The frequency of NKT cells in colon submucosa of the recipients. n=8, **, $p<0.01$, vs. WT→WT; #, $p<0.05$, vs. ApoE-/-→WT. D. The frequency of $\gamma\delta$T cells in colon submucosa of the recipients. n=8, **, $p<0.01$, vs. WT→WT; #, $p<0.05$, vs. ApoE-/-→WT. E. Average tumor number per mouse in the recipients. n=12, *, $p<0.05$, vs. WT→WT; #, $p<0.05$, vs. ApoE-/-→WT. F. Histopathologic stages of tumors. n=12, *, $p<0.05$, **, $p<0.01$ vs. WT→WT; #, $p<0.05$, ##, $p<0.01$, vs. ApoE-/-→WT [13].*

by hypercholesterolemia. As anticipated, we found hypermethylation of Fyn, Sox13, Il15R, IKT and SH2D1a in HSCs from hypercholesterolemic mice (**Figure 12B**).

As expected, the overexpression of Tet1 in HSCs from WT and ApoE−/− mice decreased the methylation and increased the expression of these five genes (**Figures 12B** and **13B**). In addition to these five genes, an additional five genes, ETV5, EGR2, SLAMF1, ZBTB16, and RELB, whose expression was unaffected in HSCs from ApoE−/− mice, nonetheless their expression increased after Tet1 overexpression (**Figure 13A**). Both NKT and γδ T are being evaluated intensely as cell immunotherapies for a variety of cancers. This opens the possibility of a combined cell therapy directed by Tet1 overexpression in HSCs.

The methylation of ETV5, EGR2, and NFKB1was higher in HSCs derived from ApoE−/− mice than in HSCs from WT mice, but overexpression of Tet1 reduced this methylation at or below that in WT HSCs (**Figure 13B**) Taken together, all of these results show that Tet1regulates the expression of multiple genes that are essential to produce NKT and γδ T cells and this regulation is disrupted by hypercholesterolemia.

2.8 Tet1 regulates histone modifications by the O-linked N-acetylglucosamine transferase (OGT)

O-linked N-acetylglucosamine transferase is an evolutionarily conserved enzyme whose primary function is to catalyze)-linked protein glycosylation. Tet2 and Tet3

Genes related to NKT cell differentiation	Genes related to γδ T cell differentiation
Interleukin-2 receptor β (IL-2Rb)	B-cell lymphoma/leukemia 11B (BCL11b)
Interleukin-15 receptor (IL-15R)	Early growth response protein 2 (EGR2)
E26 Transformation specific transcription factor 1 (Ets1)	Ets variant 5 (ETV5)
Myeloid Elf-1-like factor (MEF)	Inhibitor of DNA binding protein 2 (ID2)
Interferon regulatory factor 1 (IRF-1)	Inhibitor of DNA binding protein 3 (ID3)
Fyn	Interleukin-2-inducible T-cell kinase (ITK)
Interleukin-2-inducible T-cell kinase (Itk)	Interleukin 7 receptor (IL-7R)
Activator protein-1 (AP-1)	Interleukine-15 receptor (IL-15R)
T cell factor 1 (TCF-1)	PHD finger protein 1 (PHF1)
Nuclear factor κB p50 (NFκb)	SLAM-Associated Protein (SAP, SH2D1a)
RELb	*Sry*-related HMG box 13 (Sox13)
IκB kinase 2 (IKK2)	T cell factor 12 (TCF12)
Protein kinase C-θ (PKCθ)	Zinc finger and BTB domain-containing protein 16 (ZBTB16)
Signaling lymphocytic activation molecule F1 (SLAMF1)	
Signaling lymphocytic activation molecule-associated protein (SAP)	
Krüppel-like factor 2 (KLF2)	
CCR9	

Table 1.
The genes related to the differentiation of NKT and γδ T cells. The genes highlighted with green color showed significant changes in our study.

have been shown to act as stable partners if OGT in the nucleus [28–30]. Their interaction with OGT induces GlcNAcylation of Host Cell Factor-1 that enhances the H3K4 methyltransferase SET1/COMPASS complex, indicating that Tet enzymes increase H3K4me3 modifications that result in transcriptional activation [31]. Our immunoprecipitation results establish that OGT interacts with Tet1 in HSCs (**Figure 14A**). This Tet1-OGT interaction was significantly less in HSCs from hypercholesterolemic mice, consistent with the decrease in Tet1 expression. Overexpression of Tet1 enhanced the Tet1-OGT interaction but had no effect on the expression or interaction of Tet3 and OGT (**Figure 14A** and **B**). As anticipated by these findings, overexpression increased H3K4me3-induced methylation at the promoters of all of the genes evaluated except RELb and NFKB1. These findings indicate that Tet1's interaction with OGT increases H3K4me3 levels that help maintain an active chromatin structure near many of the genes required to produce NKT and γδ T cells by HSCs (**Figure 14C**). These results show that Tet1 regulates the expression of multiple genes required for NKT and γδ T cells by multiple mechanisms.

2.9 Hypercholesterolemia reduces Tet1 expression in human HSCs that impairs their production of NKT and γδ T cells

To determine if the effects of hypercholesterolemia on murine HSCs can be extrapolated to human HSCs, we exposed human HSCs to oxidized-LDL, the source of oxidant stress in HSCs from hypercholesterolemic mice [19].

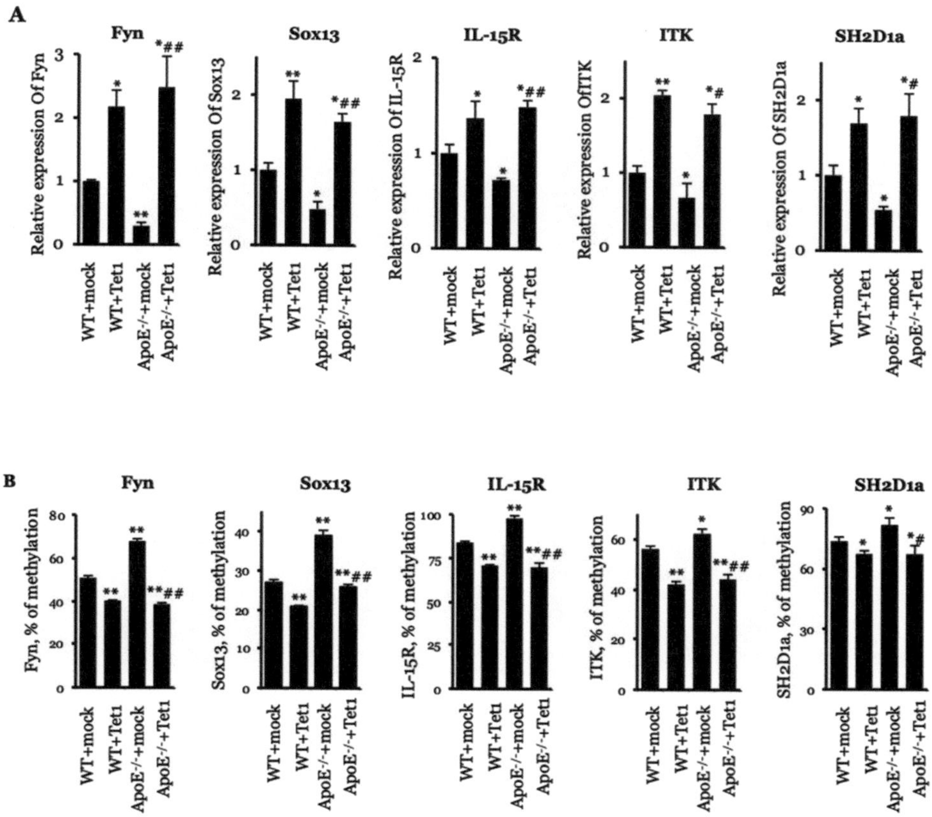

Figure 12.
*Tet1 regulates the expression of the key regulatory genes in the differentiation of NKT and γδT cells. A. The expression of genes in cells from in vitro co-culture with WT HSCs, ApoE-/- HSCs, Tet1 overexpressing WT HSCs or Tet1 overexpressing ApoE-/- HSCs. n=4, *, p<0.05, **, p<0.01, vs. WT+mock; #, p<0.05, ##, p<0.01, vs. ApoE-/-+mock. B. DNA methylation status of the targeted gene. n=4, *, p<0.05, **, p<0.01, vs. WT+mock; #, p<0.05, ##, p<0.01, vs. ApoE-/-+mock [13].*

Oxidized-LDL induced a concentration-dependent decrease in the expression of Tet1 (**Figure 15C**). This reduction in Tet1 expression reduced the differentiation of human HSCs toward NKT and γδ T cells (**Figure 15A** and **B**). These preliminary results suggest that the extensive findings from these studies are generalizable to humans.

3. Conclusions

For those under 50 years of age, CRC is the leading cause of cancer death in men and the second leading cause of death in women. More than 50% of cases are due to lifestyle risk factors. Obesity will soon replace tobacco abuse as the most preventable cause of cancer and is a significant risk for CRC. However, obesity is associated with multiple metabolic abnormalities, including hypercholesterolemia, which is a well-defined risk factor for CRC. We have shown that hypercholesterolemia impairs immunosurveillance against colorectal neoplasia by reducing the number and function of NKT and γδ T cells. In support of this role for NKT and γδ T cells in CRC

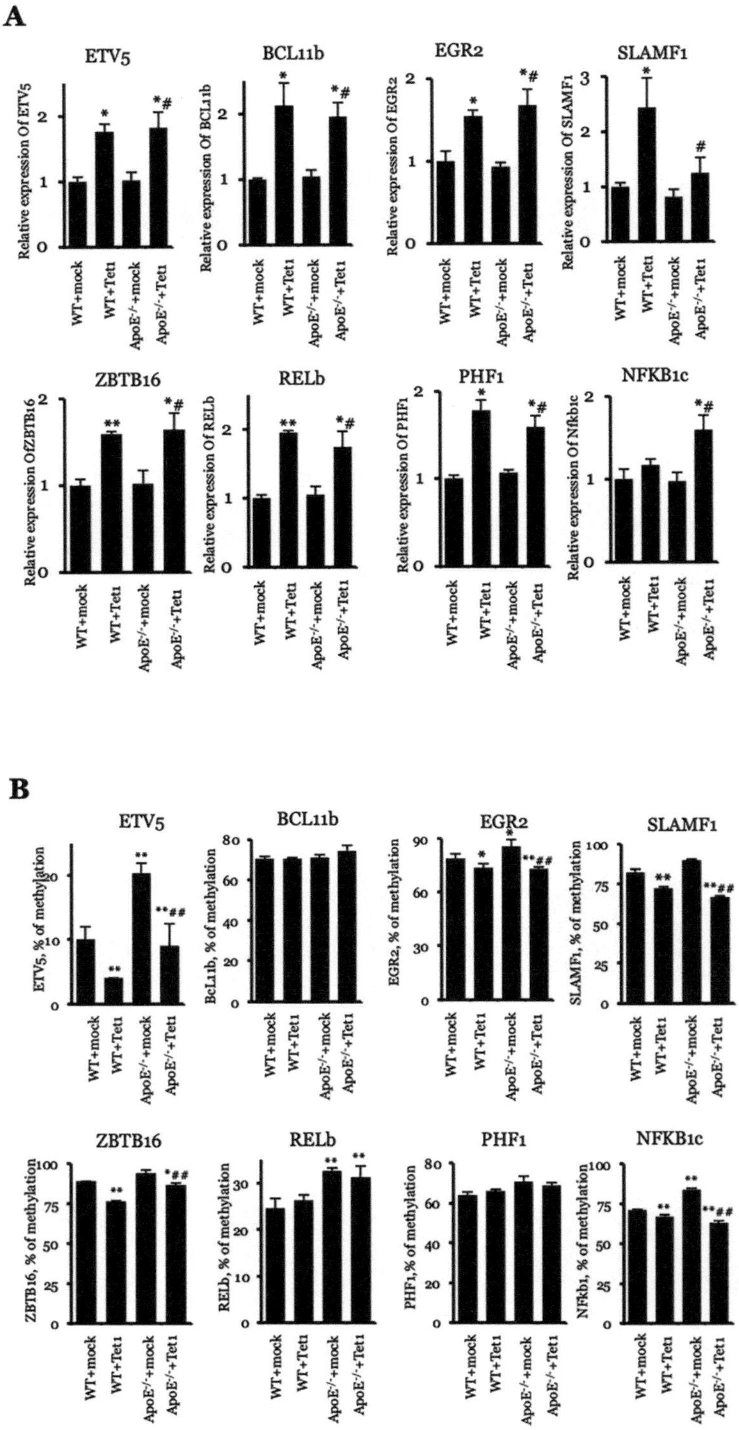

Figure 13.
*In HSCs, Tet1 overexpression reduces the expression of the key regulatory genes in their differentiation of NKT and γδT cells. A. Gene expression analysis in WT HSCs, ApoE-/- HSCs, Tet1 overexpressing WT HSCs and Tet1 overexpressing ApoE-/- HSCs. n=4, *, p<0.05, **, p<0.01, vs. WT+mock; #, p<0.05, ##, p<0.01, vs. ApoE-/-+mock. B. DNA methylation status of the genes analyzed in A. n=4, *, p<0.05, **, p<0.01, vs. WT+mock; #, p<0.05, ##, p<0.01, vs. ApoE-/-+mock [13].*

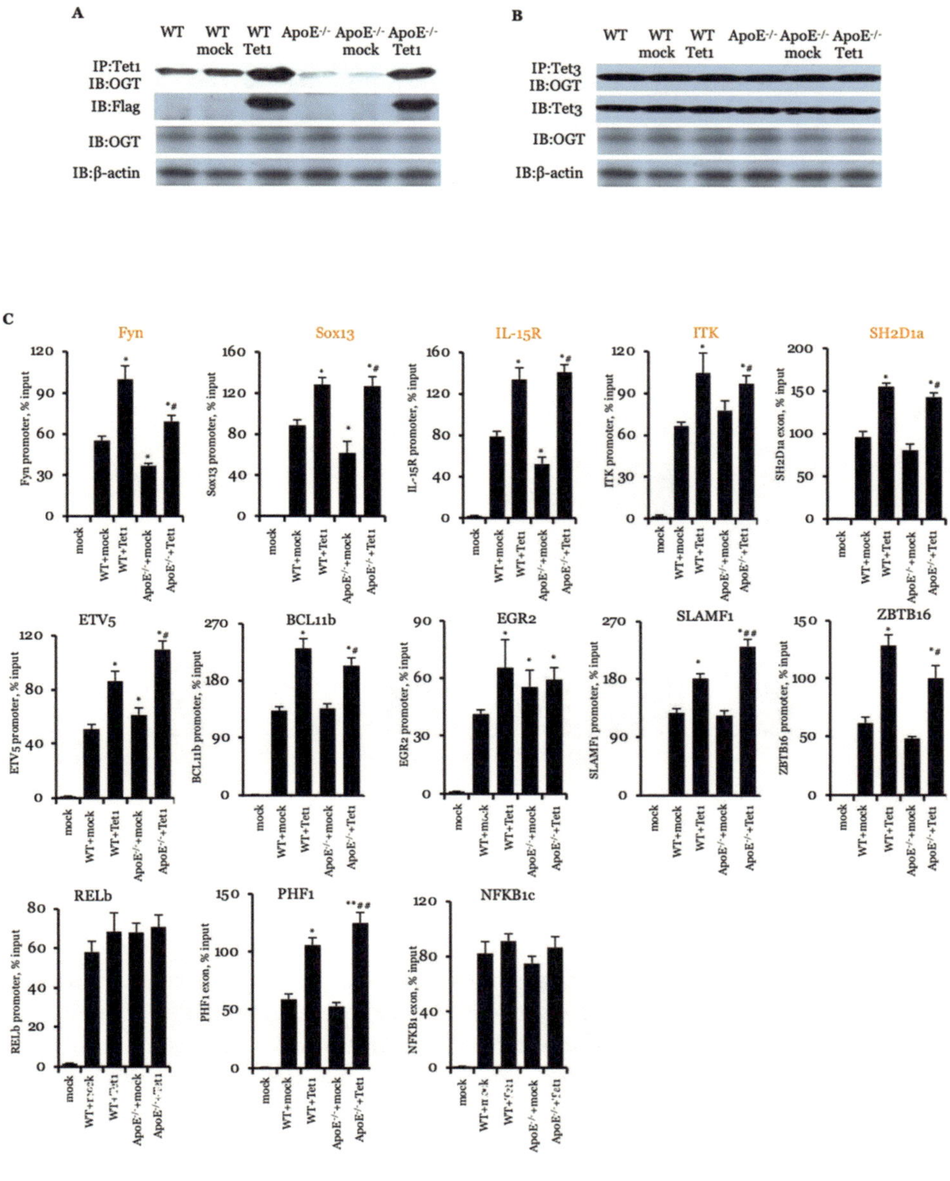

Figure 14.
*Tet1 regulates H3K4me3 modification of the key regulatory genes in the differentiation of HSCs towards NKT and γδT cells in vitro. A. Detection of the expression of Tet1 and its association with OGT. Immunoprecipitation was performed with WT HSCs, ApoE-/- HSCs, Tet1 overexpressing WT HSCs or Tet1 overexpressing ApoE-/- HSCs. B. Detection of the expression of Tet3 and its association with OGT. C. H3K4me3 modification of the key regulatory genes in the differentiation of HSCs towards NKT and γδT cells in vitro. n=4, *, p<0.05, **, p<0.01, vs. WT+mock; #, p<0.05, ##, p<0.01, vs. ApoE-/-+mock [13].*

immunosurveillance, mice lacking NKT T cells have very substantial increases in colorectal neoplasia.

At a molecular level, hypercholesterolemia induces an oxidized-LDL increase in HSC oxidant stress that initiates a signaling pathway culminating in the downregulation of Tet1whihc is directly regulated by miR101c. These effects of hypercholesterolemia on CRC are not due to a direct effect on NKT and γδ T cells, as is universally

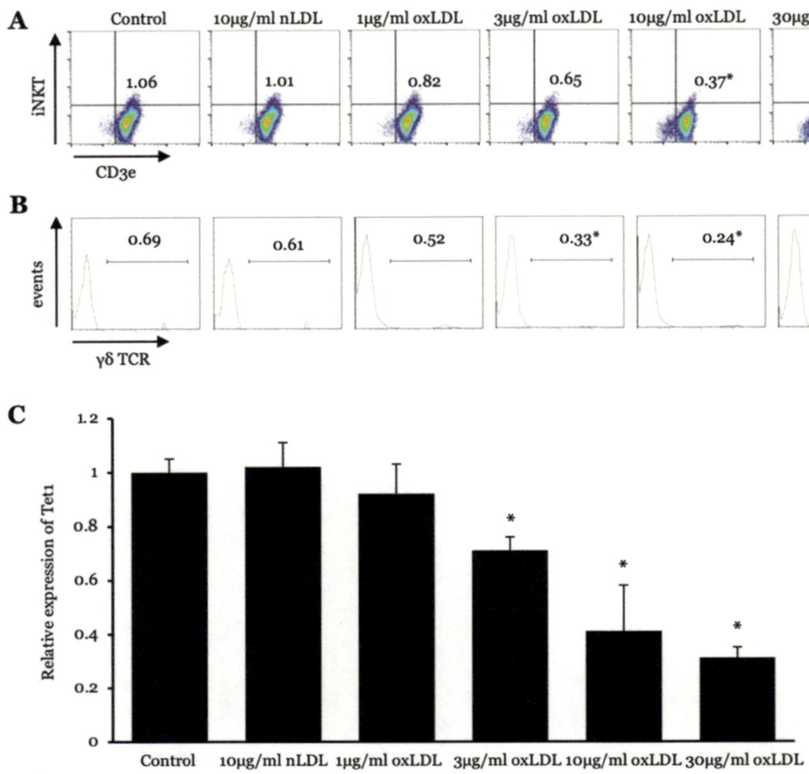

Figure 15.
*Ox-LDL impairs the differentiation of human HSCs towards NKT and γδT cells in vitro. A. Differentiation of human HSCs towards iNKT cells in vitro. B. Differentiation of human HSCs towards γδT cells in vitro. C. Relative expression of Tet1 in human HSCs treated with oxLDL. n=3, *, $p<0.05$, vs. control [13].*

held. Rather, hypercholesterolemia increases the incidence of CRC by a Tet-1dependent HSC-autonomous mechanism that epigenetically reprograms their gene expression within the HSC. This reduction in gene expression is achieved by bivalent regulation comprised of a gain of repressive DNA methylation and loss of activating H3K4me3. Thus, we show for the first time that HSCs not only produce immune cells, but they can also regulate their gene expression by oxidant stress-dependent epigenetic reprogramming.

Tet1 is a critical tumor suppressor in multiple human cancers, including colorectal cancer [32]. The analysis of tumor methylomes of tumor cell lines and primary tumors of multiple carcinomas and lymphomas, including gastric and colorectal carcinomas, showed that Tet1 is frequently methylated and consequently downregulated [33–35]. The overexpression of the Tet1 catalytic domain can significantly reduce the methylation of tumor suppressor genes and thereby restore their expression [34]. Reduced Tet1 expression can repress the expression of the DKK gene and the activation of the WNT pathway, which increases tumorigenesis in the colon. In contrast, restoring Tet1 expression in colon carcinoma cells inhibits their proliferation as well as tumor xenografts [35]. All of these studies strongly indicate that Tet1 plays a critical role in the transformation of colon cells. So, in addition to these findings, we show that Tet1 regulates the production of NKT and γδ T cells that is central to immunosurveillance against colorectal neoplasia.

Are these findings generalizable? We have also shown that type 2 diabetes mellitus (T2DM) impairs wound healing by an HSC-autonomous mechanism [36]. In parallel to our findings with hypercholesterolemia, T2DM induced a Nox-2-dependent increase in HSC oxidant stress that initiated a signaling pathway that culminated in the increased expression of Dnmt1 by reduced expression of let-7-3p. These changes reduced the expression of Klf4, Notch-1and Pu.1, genes critical to the production of monocytes and macrophages. Consequently, across the first two stages of wound healing, T2DM reduced the number of macrophages and increased their polarization toward the M-1 phenotype. Reconstituting T2DM mice with HSCs from T2DM in which an shRNA against Dnmt1 restored a normal rate of wound healing. Thus, this may be a framework to identify the mechanism of the other risk factors for young-onset CRC may be evaluated. Each risk factor induces a risk factor-specific HSC oxidant stress that initiates a signaling pathway culminating in the changed expression of an epigenetic enzyme(s) that is directly regulated by a miRNA. In this way, risk factors affect the gene expression by inducing redox-dependent epigenetic reprogramming of their gene expression within the hematopoietic stem cell.

Author details

Louis Messina[1*] and Guodong Tie[2]

1 University of Massachusetts Medical School, Worcester, MA, USA

2 Dana Farber Cancer Institute, Harvard Medical School, Boston, USA

*Address all correspondence to: louis.messina@umassmemorial.org

References

[1] Siegel RL, Giaquinto AN, Jemal A. Cancer statistics, 2024. CA: A Cancer Journal for Clinicians. 2024;**74**(1):12-49

[2] Spaander MCW, Zauber AG, Syngal S, Blaser MJ, Sung JJ, You YN, et al. Young-onset colorectal cancer. Nature Reviews. Disease Primers. 2023;**9**(1):21

[3] Francescangeli F, De Angelis ML, Zeuner A. Dietary factors in the control of gut homeostasis, intestinal stem cells, and colorectal cancer. Nutrients. 2019;**11**(12):2936

[4] O'Keefe SJ, Li JV, Lahti L, et al. Fat, fibre and cancer risk in African Americans and rural Africans. Nature Communications. 2015;**6**(1):6342

[5] Zheng X, Hur J, Nguyen LH, et al. Comprehensive assessment of diet quality and risk of precursors of early-onset colorectal cancer. Journal of the National Cancer Institute. 2021;**113**(5):543-552

[6] Koene RJ, Prizment AE, Blaes A, Konety SH. Shared risk factors in cardiovascular disease and cancer. Circulation. 2016;**133**:1104-1114

[7] Hennekens CH, Andreotti F. Leading avoidable cause of premature deaths worldwide: Case for obesity. The American Journal of Medicine. 2013;**126**:97-98

[8] Ulaganathan V, Kandiah M, Shariff ZM. A case-control study on the association of abdominal obesity and hypercholesterolemia with the risk of colorectal cancer. Journal of Carcinogenesis. 2018;**17**:4

[9] Font-Burgada J, Sun B, Karin M. Obesity and cancer: The oil that feeds the flame. Cell Metabolism. 2016;**23**:48-62

[10] Notarnicola M, Altomare DF, Correale M, Ruggieri E, D'Attoma B, Mastrosimini A, et al. Serum lipid profile in colorectal cancer patients with and without synchronous distant metastases. Oncology. 2005;**68**:371-374

[11] Zhang L, Cao F, Zhang G, Shi L, Chen S, Zhang Z, et al. Trends in and predictions of colorectal cancer incidence and mortality in China from 1990 to 2025. Frontiers in Oncology. 2019;**9**:98

[12] Jun SY, Brown AJ, Chua NK, Yoon JY, Lee JJ, Yang JO, et al. Reduction of squalene epoxidase by cholesterol accumulation accelerates colorectal cancer progression and metastasis. Gastroenterology. 2021;**160**(4):1194-1207.e1128

[13] Tie G, Yan J, Khair L, Messina JA, Deng A, Kang J, et al. Hypercholesterolemia increases colorectal cancer incidence by reducing production of NKT and gamma-DeltaT cells from hematopoietic stem cells. Cancer Research. 2017;**77**:2351-2362

[14] Lee JW, You NY, Kim Y, Kim Y, Kim J, Kang HT. Statin use and site-specific risk of colorectal cancer in individuals with hypercholesterolemia from the National Health Insurance Service-National Health Screening Cohort (NHIS-HEALS). Nutrition, Metabolism, and Cardiovascular Diseases. 2019;**29**(7):701-709

[15] van Galen P, Kreso A, Wienholds E, Laurenti E, Eppert K, Lechman ER, et al. Reduced lymphoid lineage priming promotes human hematopoietic stem cell expansion. Cell Stem Cell. 2014;**14**:94-106

[16] Guo G, Luc S, Marco E, Lin TW, Peng C, Kerenyi MA, et al. Mapping

cellular hierarchy by single-cell analysis of the cell surface repertoire. Cell Stem Cell. 2013;**13**:492-505

[17] Mercer EM, Lin YC, Benner C, Jhunjhunwala S, Dutkowski J, Flores M, et al. Multilineage priming of enhancer repertoires precedes commitment to the B and myeloid cell lineages in hematopoietic progenitors. Immunity. 2011;**35**:413-425

[18] Orkin SH. Priming the hematopoietic pump. Immunity. 2003;**19**:633-634

[19] Tie G, Messina KE, Yan J, Messina JA. Messina LM, Hypercholesterolemia induces oxidant stress that accelerates the ageing of hematopoietic stem cells. Journal of the American Heart Association. 2014;**3**:e000241

[20] Taniguchi M, Seino K, Nakayama T. The NKT cell system: Bridging innate and acquired immunity. Nature Immunology. 2003;**4**:1164-1165

[21] Todaro M, D'Asaro M, Caccamo N, Iovino F, Francipane MG, Meraviglia S, et al. Efficient killing of human colon cancer stem cells by gammadelta T lymphocytes. Journal of Immunology. 2009;**182**:7287-7296

[22] Ito S, D'Alession AC, Taranova OV, Hong K, Sowers LC, Zhang Y. Role of Tet proteins in 5mC to 5hmC conversion, ES-cell self-renewal and inner cell mass specification. Nature. 2010;**466**:1129-1133

[23] Ko M, Huang Y, Jankowska AM, Pape UJ, Tahiliani M, Bandukwala HS, et al. Impaired hydroxylation of 5-methylcytosine in myeloid cancers with mutant TET2. Nature. 2010;**468**:839-843

[24] Ito S, Shen L, Dai Q, Wu SC, Collins LB, Swenberg JA, et al. Tet proteins can convert 5-methylcytosine t o 5-formylcytosine and 5-carboxylcytosine. Science. 2011;**333**:1300-1303

[25] Matsuda JL, Gapin L. Developmental program of mouse Valpha14i NKT cells. Current Opinion in Immunology. 2005;**17**:122-130

[26] Garbe A, von Boehmer H. TCR and notch synergize in alphabeta versus gammadelta lineage choice. Trends in Immunology. 2007;**28**:124-131

[27] Wu H, Zhang Y. Mechanisms and functions of Tet protein-mediated 5- methylcytosine oxidation. Genes & Development. 2011;**25**:2436-2452

[28] Vella P, Scelfo A, Jammula S, Chiacchiera F, Williams K, Cuomo A, et al. Tet proteins connect the O-linked N-acetylglucosamine transferase Ogt to chromatin in embryonic stem cells. Molecular Cell. 2013;**49**:645-656

[29] Chen Q, Chen Y, Bian C, Fujiki R, Yu X. TET2 promotes histone O- GlcNAcylation during gene transcription. Nature. 2013;**493**:561-564

[30] Shi FT, Kim H, Lu W, He Q, Liu D, Goodell MA, et al. Ten-eleven translocation 1 (Tet1) is regulated by O-linked N-acetylglucosamine transferase (Ogt) for target gene repression in mouse embryonic stem cells. The Journal of Biological Chemistry. 2013;**288**:20776-20784

[31] Deplus R, Delatte B, Schwinn MK, Defrance M, Mendez J, Murphy N, et al. TET2 and TE.T3 regulate GlcNAcylation and H3K4 methylation through OGT and SET1/COMPASS. The EMBO Journal. 2013;**32**:645-655

[32] Cimmino L, Dawlaty MM, Ndiaye-Lobry D, Yap YS, Bakogianni S, Yu Y, et al. TET1 is a tumor suppressor

of hematopoietic malignancy. Nature Immunology. 2015;**16**:653-662

[33] Chapman CG, Mariani CJ, Wu F, Meckel K, Butun F, Chuang A, et al. TET- catalyzed 5-hydroxymethylcytosine regulates gene expression in differentiating colonocytes and colon cancer. Scientific Reports. 2015;**5**:17568

[34] Li L, Li C, Mao H, Du Z, Chan WY, Murray P, et al. Epigenetic inactivation of the CpG demethylase TET1 as a DNA methylation feedback loop in human cancers. Scientific Reports. 2016;**6**:26591

[35] Neri F, Dettori D, Incarnato D, Krepelova A, Rapelli S, Maldotti M, et al. TET1 is a tumour suppressor that inhibits colon cancer growth by derepressing inhibitors of the WNT pathway. Oncogene. 2015;**34**:4168-4176

[36] Yan J, Tie G, Wang S, Tutto A, DeMarco N, Khair L, et al. Diabetes impairs wound healing by Dnmt1-dependent dysregulation of hematopoietic stem cells differentiation towards macrophages. Nature Communications. 2018;**9**(1):33

Section 2

Treatment of Colorectal Cancer

Chapter 4

Novel Therapies for Colorectal Cancers

Muriel Battaglia, Susan L. Feldt, Marcus Marable and Ardaman Shergill

Abstract

Despite improvements in colorectal cancer screening, surgical resection, and systemic treatment, colorectal cancer remains a leading cause of cancer deaths worldwide, and survival in metastatic disease remains low. Further advancements in therapeutics are thus necessary, and two new Food and Drug Administration (FDA) approvals in the U.S were seen in 2023, with trifluridine and tipiracil with bevacizumab and fruquintinib approved in previously treated metastatic colorectal cancer. In this book chapter, we summarize current standard of care, including chemotherapy and these drug recent approvals in colorectal cancer, as well as the current landscape of diverse novel therapies under investigation. Targeted therapy has been an active therapeutic approach, particularly with BRAF, HER2, and MAPK inhibition. We also summarize the current state of immunotherapy particularly utilizing checkpoint inhibition, cancer targeted vaccines, and cellular therapies within colorectal cancer. Metastatic colorectal cancer remains a poor prognosis and novel therapies are needed, and multiple classes of novel therapeutics are promising and under current investigation.

Keywords: colorectal cancer, therapeutics, targeted therapy, immunotherapy, cellular therapy

1. Introduction

Colorectal cancer is the fourth most common cancer diagnosis in the United States, behind only breast cancer in women, prostate cancer in men, and lung and bronchus cancers [1]. Worldwide, colorectal cancer is the third most commonly diagnosed at 10% of new cancer cases [2]. Colorectal cancer represents 7.8% of new cancer cases and 8.6% of all cancer deaths in the United States. About 4.1% of US men and women will be diagnosed with colorectal during their lifetime, although colorectal cancer is more common in men. The diagnosis is most often made between ages 65 and 74 at 25.5%, and the median age at diagnosis is 66 [1].

Incidence of colorectal cancer in the U.S. had been decreasing since 2000 overall and particularly in screening-aged populations above age 50. Decreasing incidence has continued to be seen in the population above 60 [3]. Declining incidence particularly in these age ranges has largely been attributed to the success of screening particularly with colonoscopy [4].

Colorectal cancer is the second most common cause of cancer death in the US [1]. Worldwide, it is also the second most common cause of cancer death at 9.4% [2]. Five-year relative survival in the United States over 2013–2019 was 65.0% [1]. This has slowly improved since the 1970s, when 5 years relative survival was 50% [5]. Despite advances in treatment, in patients with metastatic colorectal cancer, median overall survival remains low at 30 months [6].

Early- or young-onset colorectal cancer has generally been defined as diagnosis under the age of 50 years [7]. This cutoff is corresponding to the prior guidelines for initiating screening in the general average-risk population at age 50 [8]. In patients under the age of 50, the trend of incidence has been the reverse, and incidence rates are increasing [9]. This trend of declining or stable incidence above age 50 with rising incidence under age 50 has also been seen globally, in Germany, Australia, UK, Denmark, New Zealand, Canada, Slovenia, and Sweden [10].

Early-onset colorectal cancer includes those with a genetic predisposition, but this does not account for most early-onset colorectal cancer, with only about 16% having a known germline genetic variant putting them at risk [11]. The cause of this rising incidence in adults under 50 is not yet clear, but lifestyle risk factors like obesity and metabolic syndrome and alcohol consumption have been associated [7].

With rising incidence in young adults and overall survival in metastatic disease remaining low, there remains a great need for innovative treatment strategies to improve survival. Novel therapies are emerging and changing the treatment paradigm and prognosis of colorectal cancer. 2023 saw two new Food and Drug Administration (FDA) approvals in the United States for therapies in previously treated metastatic colorectal cancer; trifluridine and tipiracil with bevacizumab and fruquintinib were both approved in 2023 [11, 12]. In this article, we will summarize the current treatment paradigm in colorectal cancer including these two new approvals. We'll also then discuss the current landscape of novel emerging treatments including targeted therapies, immunotherapy with checkpoint inhibition, vaccines, and cellular therapies.

2. Immunotherapy

Immunotherapy consists of therapies that activate the patient's immune system to destroy cancerous cells. The most notable mechanism within this therapeutic category is immune checkpoint blockade which works by blocking downregulation of the immune system. This can be achieved using antibodies that target the cytotoxic T lymphocyte antigen-4 and programmed death-1 pathways. Nivolumab (PD-1 inhibitor), ipilimumab (CTLA-4 inhibitor), pembrolizumab (PD-1 inhibitor) are prominent antibodies that act as checkpoint inhibitors [13]. Checkpoint inhibitors have been studied and shown promise in numerous solid tumor types, particularly in melanoma and non-small cell lung cancer [14, 15].

In colorectal cancer, the benefit of checkpoint inhibitors has been less widespread. Most promise has been seen in tumors that are microsatellite instability-high (MSI-H) or mismatch-repair-deficient (dMMR). Microsatellites are short repeating sequences of DNA prone to error during replication which causes alteration through losses or insertions. Mismatch repair is a mechanism to recognize and repair these errors. A high number of microsatellites is then prone to error, and a deficiency in mismatch repair prevents correction of these alterations [16]. Around 15% of all colorectal cancers are dMMR, but MSI-H/dMMR is more prevalent in earlier stage tumors and the percentage of tumors that are MSI-H/dMMR declines with increasing stages [17].

This is in contrast to tumors that are mismatch repair proficient (pMMR) and microsatellite stable (MSS). The focus of checkpoint inhibitors in the MSI-H/dMMR setting came from early studies in which PD-1 inhibition as monotherapy showed anti-tumor activity in this population. Pembrolizumab was given to both patients that were dMMR/MSI-H and pMMR/MSS. In one phase II trial of patients with progressed metastatic disease, the dMMR/MSS cohort had a significantly higher ORR at 40% (95% CI 12–74), while the pMMR/MSS cohort had an ORR of 0% (95% CI 0–20). This focused following trials on dMMR/MSI-H tumors [18].

The first FDA approval of a checkpoint inhibitor in colorectal cancer was in 2017, when pembrolizumab was approved as second line treatment for metastatic colorectal cancer with microsatellite instability-high (MSI-H) tumors. This was following five clinical trials of MSI-H and dMMR tumors (with most being colorectal primaries, although other tumor types with these abnormalities were enrolled) which found an overall response rate of 39.6% (95% CI 31.7–47.9) and a 7% complete response rate [19].

Pembrolizumab was then studied in patients with metastatic MSI-H or dMMR colorectal cancer as first line treatment. In a phase 3, open-label trial, 307 patients who had not previously received treatment were randomized to pembrolizumab 200 mg every 3 weeks or chemotherapy (5-fluoruracil-based with or without bevacizumab or cetuximab) every 2 weeks. Median progression free survival (PFS) was longer with pembrolizumab than chemotherapy (16.5 vs. 8.2 months, hazard ratio 0.60; 95% CI 0.45–0.80). Grade 3 or higher treatment-related adverse events were also less common in patients who received pembrolizumab versus chemotherapy (22% and 66%, respectively) [20]. Based on these results, pembrolizumab is now FDA approved as first-line therapy for metastatic MSI-H or dMMR colorectal cancer.

Nivolumab and ipilimumab are also approved in combination in MSI-H/dMMR metastatic colorectal cancer. In the phase II CheckMate 142 trial, patients with metastatic MSI-H/dMMR colorectal cancer who had not received prior treatment received nivolumab every 2 weeks plus low-dose ipilimumab every 6 weeks until disease progression. ORR was 69% (95% CI 53–82). Grade 3 or greater treatment-related adverse events were seen in 22% of patients with 13% discontinuing treatment due to treatment-related adverse events of any grade [21].

With the success of checkpoint inhibitors in MSI-H/dMMR seen in the metastatic setting, application of checkpoint inhibitors to the adjuvant and neoadjuvant settings for earlier staged colorectal cancers is undergoing study currently. This setting may be of particular clinical benefit because a higher percentage of stage II and stage III colorectal cancers are MSI-H/dMMR compared to metastatic disease. The POLEM trial is an ongoing phase III randomized trial of avelumab (anti-PD-L1 antibody) plus fluoropyrimidine-based chemotherapy in the adjuvant setting for stage III colorectal cancer. Patients with completely resected stage III colon cancer confirmed to be dMMR/MSI-H are eligible and are randomized to standard chemotherapy or chemotherapy followed by avelumab 10 mg/kg every 2 weeks for 24 weeks. Primary end point will be disease free survival [22].

The ATOMIC trial is another ongoing phase III randomized trial of immunotherapy in the adjuvant setting for dMMR/MSI-H tumors. Patients with resected stage III colon carcinomas with dMMR/MSI-H are randomized to modified FOLFOX6 for 6 months alone or in combination with atezolizumab (anti-PD-1 antibody) at 840 mg IV every 2 weeks with chemotherapy and continuation of atezolizumab alone for an additional 6 months for a total of a year of therapy. The primary end point will also be disease free survival [23].

Numerous trials are ongoing looking back to immunotherapy in the pMMR/MSS population. As the majority of metastatic colorectal cancers are pMMR/MSS, benefit in this area would apply to a significantly higher number of patients. With limited benefit seen in monotherapy with approved checkpoint inhibitors in pMMR/MSS in early studies, current trials are more commonly utilizing checkpoint inhibitors in combination with another agent, either with chemotherapy, targeted therapies, or dual-agent immunotherapy as combination therapy.

Pembrolizumab has been studied in combination with chemotherapy in pMMR/MSS tumors. In a single-arm, phase 1b study, pembrolizumab was studied in combination with FOLFOX6 chemotherapy in metastatic colorectal adenocarcinoma regardless of mismatch repair status. A safety run-in for six patients was completed first, and grade 3 and 4 neutropenia led to dose reduction of FOLFOX6 in the expansion cohort. 30 treatment-naïve patients received combination pembrolizumab and FOLFOX. ORR was 56.7%, and median PFS was 8.8 months (80% CI 7.7–11.3). Treatment-related adverse events were limited, mainly the neutropenia seen in the safety run-in [24].

Nivolumab in combination with the VEGF inhibitor regorafenib is under investigation as well. A phase 1b trial of advanced of metastatic colon and gastric cancers refractory or intolerant to standard chemotherapy studied nivolumab plus regorafenib until disease progression or toxicity. 49 of 50 patients were pMMR/MSS. Overall ORR was 40%, with a ORR in patients with colorectal cancer of 36%. Median PFS in colorectal cancer was 7.9 months. Common grade 3 or greater treatment-related adverse events included rash (12%) and proteinuria (12%) [25]. This combination is undergoing further investigation in an ongoing phase III trial.

Two newer checkpoint inhibitors have shown some early promise in pMMR/MSS. Botensilimab is a next generation anti-CTLA-4 antibody that is under investigation in combination with balstilimab, an anti-PD-1 antibody in the pMMR/MSS setting. Results of a phase 1a/1b trial of botensilimab plus balstilimab in metastatic pMMR/MSS colorectal cancer with significant prior treatment (including 31% whom had received prior immunotherapy) were presented at ASCO GI 2023. ORR of 23% (95% CI 14–34) was seen in this cohort, and PFS was 4.1 months (95% CI 2.8–5.5). Grade 3 or greater treatment-related adverse events were seen in 43% of patients, most commonly diarrhea/colitis (21%) [26]. In two patients with locally advanced pMMR/MSS colorectal cancer, botensilimab and balstilimab were given in combination in the neoadjuvant setting. Histologically, both patients showed rapid immune response [27].

Immunotherapy is a developing therapeutic approach in numerous solid tumors, but progress in colorectal cancer has been more limited. However, success with checkpoint inhibitors in the dMMR/MSI-H population in metastatic disease has led to first line approval of pembrolizumab in this setting. Numerous trials with immunotherapy are ongoing with some promising early results, most notably in neoadjuvant and adjuvant settings for dMMR/MSI-H tumors as well as new combination therapy for the pMMR/MSS metastatic population.

3. Current therapies

Current treatments for colon cancer must be considered in the context of the tumor stage and unique genetic attributes when considering chemotherapies and biologics. Colorectal cancers are typically staged according to two systems, AJCC staging and TNM staging, which similarly take into account depth of tumor penetration, lymph node involvement, and presence of tumor metastasis [28]. For the purposes of this review, we will refer to AJCC staging when we refer to tumor stage. Stage 1 colorectal cancer, in which the tumor is localized and invades into the muscularis propria, can be managed exclusively through surgical resection, and then regular monitoring [29]. Stage 2 colorectal cancer, in which the tumor remains localized, but has penetrated into the pericolic tissue, patients can be managed with surgery with consideration for adjuvant chemotherapy for high risk patients. High risk patients as defined by having positive margins, lymphovascular invasion, poorly differentiated tumors, perineurial invasion, perforation, tumor deposits, inadequate lymph node sampling, and T4 lesions [30, 31]. For stage 3 colorectal cancer, in which the tumor has become locally advanced, with lymph nodes positive for tumor tissue, surgery and adjuvant chemotherapy is recommended [31]. Patients with Stage 4 colorectal cancer, cancers which have metastasized, are no longer considered primarily surgical candidates, with some exceptions for exclusively liver or lung metastases, and patients with acute surgical indications due to tumor location. As such, the treatment for these patients consists of chemotherapy and biologic agents (**Figure 1**) [32, 33].

The surgical approaches to colorectal cancer tumor resection consists of a transrectal and transabdominal approaches for rectal tumors, and colectomy for colon cancers. The transrectal approach is recommended only to Stage 1 tumors which make up <30% circumference of the bowel, are <3 cm in size, non fixed, and within 8 cm of the anal verge [29]. Alternatively, the transabdominal approach as a means of obtaining total mesolectal excision reduces positive margin and recurrence, and is a possibility for tumors in which transrectal approaches are not possible [34]. Both of these approaches are able to be minimally invasive, however, several studies have documented higher rates of incomplete and positive residual circumferential margins, and as such, must be considered carefully [35]. In patients with a primary tumor which is located more distally along the colon, a colectomy should be considered [36]. For colorectal cancer metastases, knowledge of location and extent of spread is pivotal. For liver metastases, hepatic resection is a possibility, but it is recommended to consider this as a consideration only if there are no unresectable extrahepatic

	TREATMENT		
STAGE	SURGERY	CHEMOTHERAPY	BIOLOGIC
STAGE 1	✔		
STAGE 2	✔	✔ 1	
STAGE 3	✔	✔	
STAGE 4	✔ 2	✔	✔

Graphic 1 Basic Colorectal Cancer Treatment Paradigm
1. For high-risk patients
2. Based on location of Metastases

Figure 1.
Basic colorectal cancer treatment paradigm. 1. For high-risk patients. 2. Based on location of metastases.

sites of tumor spread, and hepatic function can be preserved [37]. Lung metastases alternatively are eligible for resection regardless of extra pulmonary metastases, with the similar goal of maintaining native organ function, and having a primary tumor which is resectable [38]. Notably, radiation therapy can also be considered in patients with a limited number of liver or lung metastases [39].

Other surgical indications in colorectal cancer include SBO vs. signs of imminent obstruction, significant bleeding, perforation, or other tumor mass related symptoms, for these, resection, diverting ostomy, bowel bypass, and stenting can be considered [40]. Radiation therapy is a necessary consideration with respect to tumor respectability, as neoadjuvant radiation therapy with concurrent fluorpyrimide based chemotherapy can be considered in patients with non-metastatic colon cancer for the goal of achieving resectable tumors [41].

Most currently utilized chemotherapy regimens for colon cancer is based on 5-Fluorouracil (5-FU) and Leucovorin (LV), with multiple studies showing significant risk reduction in death in comparison to observation for patients with stage III colorectal cancer [42, 43]. There are now multiple chemotherapy regimens which base itself on this combination, including the biweekly infusion termed LV5FU2, the Roswell Park Schedule, and the Mayo Clinic Regimen. Researchers have looked to develop alternatives to this combination in the form of alternative fluorpyrimidines, notably capecitabine, (Xeloda) which has been found to be non inferior to 5-FU with Leucovorin [44]. Other drugs have been studied in combination with 5-FU and LV, including the addition of oxaliplatin (FOLFOX-4), which was shown to have a statistically significant improvement in 3-year disease-free survival in comparison to the cohort who received LV5FU2 [45]. Given its efficacy the FOLFOX regimen has undergone several iterations, with similar levels of efficacy and toxicity [46]. Irinotecan is a topoisomerase inhibitor which has been studied in several combinations, IFL (Irinotecan + LV + 5-FU bolus) and FOLFIRI (Irinotecan + LV + 5-FU infusion over 48 hours). While IFL has yet to show clinical benefit in comparison to 5-FU and LV in combination, and in some studies, shown inferiority, FOLFIRI has been found to improve progression-free survival [47–49]. Capecitabine and Oxaliplatin in combination, termed Xelox, has also been studied in comparison to FOLFOX-4 and 6, and shown to be non-inferior [50, 51]. To take these combinations a step further, FOLFOXIRI, combining 5-FU + LV + Irinotecan + Oxaliplat in, has been shown to improved overall response rate and of attaining complete remission, but has been shown to have greater levels of toxicity in comparison to FOLFIRI and FOLFOX [52]. Bevacizumab, an anti-VEGF monoclonal antibody, has been shown to prolong progression-free survival, when combined with 5-FU and oxaliplatin based chemotherapy for colon cancer, including IFL, XELOX, FOLFOX [53, 54], without significant increases in observed toxicities. Naturally, as a next step, FOLFOXIRI + bevacizumab was shown improves survival in comparison to FOLFOX and FOLFIRI + bevacizumab, except in patients with BRAF-mutations [55].

Advances in rectal cancer treatment have interestingly inverted the initial approach to treatment.

Instead of removing the primary tumor, and then treating with chemotherapy, the approach is to now treat with chemotherapy, coupled or followed by radiation therapy or chemoradiotherapy, surgical intervention, followed by adjuvant chemotherapy. Total Neoadjuvant Therapy (TNT), which consists of treating a patient with systemic chemotherapy and radiotherapy prior to consideration of surgical intervention, has been shown to result in lower rates of metastases, lower rates of disease-related treatment failure, and had higher rates of pathological complete response [56].

Notably, this trial failed to show a change in 3-year survival. Neoadjuvant chemotherapy regimens are similar to those of colon cancer. FOLFOX, has been shown to have a significant effect on progression-free survival in patients with colon and rectal cancer, 9 vs. 6.2 months [57]. As for the agents utilized for chemoradiotherapy, Capecitabine, and 5-FU have been shown to be efficacious in the treatment of locally advanced rectal cancer, including achieving complete clinical remissions in a small number of patients, capecitabine being preferred due to side effect profile [58]. Chemoradiotherapy being preformed prior to surgical intervention was supported by the results of the CAO/ARO/AIO-12 trials, which compared preoperative vs. postoperative chemoradiotherapy for rectal cancer. This trial demonstrated that local recurrence was significantly lower in patients who receive preoperative chemoradiotherapy vs. patients who received postoperative chemoradiotherapy [59]. TNT with mFOLFIRINOX was studied in the PRODIGE 23 trial, which showed that patients who received this therapy prior to chemoradiotherapy, surgery, and adjuvant chemotherapy with FOLFOX, had improved 5-year survival, overall survival, metastatic-free survival in comparison to patients who did not receive the mFOLFIRINOX, but received all other interventions [60].

Metastatic colorectal cancer treatments can be considered grouped to some degree. 5-FU, capecitabine, oxalliplatin, irinotecan, and bevacizumab remain acceptable treatments, with other chemotherapeutics, biologics, and immunotherapies being considered. See **Figure 2** for an overall guideline regarding first to fourth line treatments for metastatic CRC grouped by their genetic profile.

Biologic agents for metastatic colon cancer can be grouped by their pathways, broadly vascular endothelial growth factor (VEGF) and epidermal growth factor receptor (EGFR). Aflibercept, a fusion protein of two VEGF receptors extracellular domains (VEGFR1 and VEGFR2), was shown to improve overall survival when added to FOLFIRI in comparison patients with metastatic colorectal cancer who exclusively received FOLFIRI [61]. Ramucirumab, a monoclonal antibody which targets the VEGFR2 extracellular domain, similarly showed an improvement in the overall survival of patients when added to FOLFIRI in patients with metastatic colorectal cancer [62]. Cetuximab, a mouse/human chimeric monoclonal antibody against EGFR, was

	RAS MUTANT	RAS/BRAF V600E WILDTYPE, HER2 NEG	BRAF V600E MUTATED	HER2 OVEREXPRESSION
FIRST LINE	• Doublet therapy • Triplet therapy w/ Anti-VEGFi	• Left: Doublet with anti-EGFR • Right: doublet or triplet therapy with anti-VEGFi	• Doublet therapy • Triplet therapy with anti-VEGFi	• Doublet therapy • Triplet therapy with anti-VEGFi
SECOND LINE	• Doublet therapy with anti-VEGFi	• Doublet with anti-VEGFi	• Encorafinib-cetuximab	• Doublet with anti-VEGFi
THIRD LINE	• Regorafinib • Lonsurf +/- Bevacizumab • Fruquitinib	• anti-EGFR +/- irinotecan	• Doublet with anti-VEGFi	• Transtuzumab with pertuzumab or lapatinib • fam-transtuzumab deruxtecan
FOURTH LINE		• Regorafinib • Lonsurf+/-Bev • Fruquintinib • Anti-EGFR rechallenge	• Regorafinib • Lonsurf+/-Bev • Fruquintinib	• Regorafinib • Lonsurf+/-Bev • Fruquintinib

Figure 2.
Immunotherapy for MSI-H/d-MMR cancers.

shown to improve overall survival from 4.6 to 6.1 months, and improve progression-free survival when compared to supportive care [63]. Panitumumab, a human mAB against EGFR, has been shown to improve overall survival when added to mFOLFOX6 regimens in patients with RAS wild-type left-sided metastatic colorectal cancer who had received no prior chemotherapy in comparison to those patients that were treated with mFOLFOX6 + bevacizumab [64]. Regorafenib, a tyrosine kinase inhibitor which was shown in the CORRECT trial to improve overall survival (6.4 vs. 5 months) when compared to placebo in patients with refractory metastatic colorectal cancer [65]. Pembrolizumab, an anti PD-1 mAB, was compared to 5-FU based regimens (FOLFOX or FOLFIRI) alone or with bevacizumab vs. cetuximab in patients with MSI-H metastatic colorectal cancers, and found to prolong progression free survival [20]. Nivolumab, another anti PD-1 mAB, has been shown to have achieved disease control in a statically significant disease control in patients with treatment MSI-H metastatic colorectal cancer [66]. Encorafinib, a kinase inhibitor which targets BRAF V600E, has been shown prolong survival when combined with cetuximab and binimetinib in patients with BRAF V600E-mutated colorectal cancer, when compared to first line chemotherapy [66]. Notably, two new treatments for metastatic colorectal cancer were approved in 2023, the combination of trifluoride and tipiracil (termed lonsurf) with bevacizumab and fruquitinib. Lonsurf with bevacizumab was compared to Lonsurf alone was shown to lengthen median overall survival in patients with metastatic colorectal cancer [67]. Fruquitinib was compared to placebo in patients with refractory metastatic colorectal cancer, and was found similarly to lengthen median overall survival [68].

4. Vaccine

Vaccines as a method of preventing initial occurrence, inhibiting tumor progression, promoting treatment response, and preventing recurrence have been an area of increased interest for multiple types of cancer [69]. Despite theoretical benefit and promising studies showing improved survival and recurrence rates, there are no approved vaccines for any colorectal cancer subtype [69]. The antigens which cancer vaccines can target include tumor-associated antigens (TAAs), proteins present on normal and tumor cells, but are typically over expressed on tumor cells, and tumor-specific antigens (TSAs), which are present only on tumor cells. TSA targeting vaccines would be beneficial in that these vaccines would have more direct activity with fewer systemic effects. Beyond their target proteins, cancer vaccines can be further subdivided by their vector of transmission.

Peptide based vaccines contain epitopes of the TAAs and TSAs targets, are presented to the patient's T-cells by antigen presenting cells via the major histocompatibility complex eliciting an immune response against the target [70]. As opposed to presenting the antigens, DNA and mRNA based vaccines, deliver genetic information to have cells produce and target TAAs and TSAs through various mechanisms.

Viruses, bacteria, and yeast based vaccinations all seek to take advantage of a patient's native immune mechanisms. These vaccines express TAA and TSA transgenes, for the goal of promoting pathogen-associated molecular to trigger an immune response against the target [71, 72]. Notable distinctions between these vectors, include viral vectors ability to target specific antigen-presenting cells [73]. Bacterial vectors induce a cell-mediated and humoral immune responses, with some bacteria targeting solid tumors preferentially due of the tumor microenvironment [74]. Of the yeast species typically utilized for yeast based vaccines, they are considered safe given

Phase	Brief description	ClinicalTrials ID
I	Safety, dosing, and efficacy of a personalized neoepitope yeast-based vaccine in patients s/p curative treatment for several types of solid cancers.	NCT03552718
II	Efficacy of MUC1 peptide-poly-ICLC adjuvant vaccine in patient's with newly diagnosed advanced adenomatous polyps.	NCT02134925
I/II	Safety and efficacy of galinpepimut-S vaccine with pembrolizumab in several types of advanced cancers.	NCT03761914
II	Efficacy of CV301 vaccine in combination with multiple drugs in patients with metastatic and recurrent small bowl and CRCs.	NCT04491955
II/III	Effect on ctDNA of Maintenance Therapy with GRT-C901/GRT-R902 vaccines in combination with checkpoint inhibitors + Fluorpyrimidine and Bevacizumab vs. Fluoropyrimidine and Bevacizumab alone.	NCT05141721
I/II	Safety and efficacy of frameshift-derived neoantigen dendritic cell vaccination on subjects with dMMR CRC and carriers of MMR-gene mutation without signs of CRC	NCT01885702
I/II	Safety and efficacy of NANT CRC vaccine vs. Regorafenib in patients with Metastatic CRC s/p SOC treatment	NCT03563157
II	Safety and efficacy of PolyPEPI1018 vaccine and atezolizumab in patients with MSS CRC who have progressed s/p 2/3 SOC regimens.	NCT05243862

Table 1.
Collection of all currently active clinical trials documented in ClinicalTrials.gov *for cancer vaccines in CRC patients. January 2023.*

their non-pathogenic nature [75]. There are also vaccines which use dendritic cells as a vector. Dendritic cells, function as antigen presenting cells, and when used as vaccines, trigger T cell activity directly [76]. These cells can be taken directly from the patient, cultured, modified, and expanded, prior to being re-infused into the patient. These cells can be modified by being mixed with TAAs and TSAs, tumor cell lysates, or exposed to a viral vector in order to express the protein target. Active studies into vaccines for colorectal cancer are looking into a variety of the above topics (**Table 1**).

5. Cell directed therapy

Cellular directed therapy, in which genetically modified immune cells are primed to target tumor cells has been a growing area of interest. Showing significant promise in the treatment of hematological cancers, many researchers are seeking to demonstrate efficacy in solid tumors, particularly colorectal cancer (**Table 2**). There have been multiple approaches to cell directed therapy developed, with the major ones being categorized as tumor-infiltrating lymphocytes (TILs), natural killer cells, cytokine-induced killer cells, chimeric antigen receptor (CAR) T cells, and engineered T cell receptors (TCR).

When using tumor-infiltrating lymphocytes (TILs) researchers isolate and extract lymphocytes which have infiltrated tumor, they are then amplified and then reintroduced into the patient. Given that these cells have not been modified during this process, less reactions are expected in comparison to alternative treatments, but notably, TILs efficacy is limited by tumors inherent immunosuppressive microenvironment [77]. Natural killer (NK) cells, innate lymphocytes which directly target tumors, have

Phase	Brief description	ClinicalTrials ID
II	Safety and efficacy of Cytokine-Induced Killer Cells + S-1 and Bevacizumab S-1 and Bevacizumab alone as maintenance treatment for Stage 4 CRC.	NCT02487992
I	Safety of anti-HER2 CAR Macrophages in patients with all HER2 over-expressing solid tumors	NCT04660929
I	Safety of an infusion of CD39+ and CD103+ tumor infiltrating lymphocytes among patients with multiple tumor types.	NCT05902520
II	Efficacy of autologous expanded tumor infiltrating lymphocytes amount subjects with multiple tumor types.	NCT03610490
I	Safety and efficacy of LYL845 (a tumor infiltrating lymphocyte) in patients with melanoma, NSCLC, and CRC.	NCT05573035
I	Safety of TBio-4101, a neoantigen-selected, TIL with pembrolizomab +/− SOC chemotherapy and RT in patients with advanced solid malignancies.	NCT05576077
II	Efficacy of short-term cultured TILs with Pembrolizomab following SOC in subjects with metastatic solid cancers	NCT01174121
II	Efficacy of TIL with high dose aldesleukin in patients with advanced, recurrent, or metastatic solid cancers.	NCT03935893
I	Safety of NKG2D CAR-T therapy in patients with previously treated liver metastatic CRC infused by hepatic artery.	NCT05248048
I	Safety of NKG2D CAR-NK therapy in patients with refractory metastatic CRC administered by intra-peritoneal infusion, then by IV, with a plan to include other cancer types.	NCT05213195
I/II	Safety and efficacy of NKT cells in patients with unresectable advanced solid tumors.	NCT02562963
I	Safety of anti-HER2 oNK cells in patients with advanced or metastatic HER2-expressing cancer types.	NCT04319757
I	Safety of CYAD 101(allogenic chimeric antigen Receptor t-cells) administered with FOLFOX followed by pembrolizumab in patients with unresectable metastatic colorectal cancer.	NCT04991948
I	Safety of CYAD 101(allogenic chimeric antigen Receptor t-cells) after FOLFOX or FOLFIRI therapy in patients with unresectable metastatic colorectal cancer	NCT03692429
I/II	Safety and efficacy of CNA3103 (LGR5 targeted CAR T-cells) in patients with metastatic CRC.	NCT05759728
I	Safety of GCC19CART in patients with relapsed or refractory metastatic CRC.	NCT05319314
I	Safety and efficacy of IM96 CAR-T (anti-GUCY2C) cells in patients with advanced digestive system neoplasms.	NCT05287165
I	Safety of HER2-specific CAR T-cells with CAdVEC (an oncolytic adenovirus) in HER2 positive solid tumors	NCT03740256
I/II	Safety and efficacy of A2B530 (autologous logic-gated Tmod CAR T-cells) in patient's with recurrent, unresectable, advanced, or metastatic solid tumors, all with CEA expression and are gremlin HLA-A*02 heterogeneous.	NCT05736731
I	Safety of P-MUC1C-ALLO1 (Mucin1 targeting CAR T-cell) with Rimiducid in patients with advanced or metastatic epithelial derived solid tumors.	NCT05239143
I	Safety of EpCAM targeting CAR T-cells. In patients with malignant digestive system tumors.	NCT05028933

Phase	Brief description	ClinicalTrials ID
I	Safety of anti-CEA CAR T-cells in patients with CEA + CRC metastatic to the liver with minimal residual lesions postoperatively.	NCT05240950
I	Safety of anti-CEA CAR T-cells in patients with CEA + advanced malignant solid tumors.	NCT06043466 NCT05415475 NCT05396300 NCT04348643
I	Safety of αPD1-MSLN-CAR T-cells (Mesothelin targeting) in patients with MSLN positive advanced solid tumors.	NCT05089266

Table 2.
Collection of all currently active clinical trials documented in ClinicalTrials.gov *for cell directed therapy in CRC patients. January 2023.*

also been an area of research. Endogenous NK cells are similarly extracted and amplified, but also undergo genetic modification to allow them to promote their anti-tumor activity, and improve their drug resistance [78]. Cytokine-induced killer cell therapy, in which CD3+CD56+ and CD3CD56- lymphocytes are extracted and amplified ex vivo, and exposed to cytokines (i.e., IL-12, IL-15, and IL-18) in order to maintain their anti-tumor activity in the absence of antibody detection when they are reintroduced into the patient [79]. Chimeric antigen receptor (CAR) T cells, T cells which have had a retroviral vector introduce a chimeric antigen receptor, allowing these T cells to now target the protein of interest. While results have been promising, adoption has been limited due to cost, and life-threatening toxicities [78, 80]. Engineered or cloned T cell receptors (TCR) cells function similarly to CAR T cells, but instead have had the vector introduce T cell receptors which bind to major histocompatibility complexes known to be associated with certain TAAs and TSAs [81]. As such, TCR cells are not limited to cell surface antigens like CAR T cells.

6. Targeted therapies

Targeted therapies for colorectal cancer are a rapidly expanding and effective approach to advanced cases, particularly metastatic disease. These therapies work by modifying fundamental cell processes—including growth and migration—as well as promoting host immune response against cancer cells [82].

Targeted therapies include mitogen-activated protein kinase (MAPK) inhibitors, human epidermal growth factor receptor two (HER2) inhibitors, and BRAF gene inhibitors, among others and among an evolving landscape of gene targets. Choice of targeted therapy depends on tumor-specific molecular factors and the stage and progression of the cancer [83].

6.1 MAPK inhibitors

MAPK inhibitors encompass multiple proteins involved in epidermal growth factor (EGF) cellular pathways, a growth factor that is frequently overexpressed in colorectal cancers. They also serve to enhance the inflammatory response and anti-tumor immunity [84]. These proteins include extracellular-signal-regulated kinases (ERK MAPK), the c-jun N-terminal kinase (JNK), stress-activated protein kinases (SAPK), and mitogen-activated protein kinase 14 (MAPK14) [85].

Examples of commonly utilized MAPK inhibitors include Trametinib and Cobimetinib, which—by inhibiting the MEK protein, a downstream mediator of RAS in the MAPK pathway—impede cancer cell growth and proliferation [86]. These agents are often used in combination with a BRAF gene inhibitor in cases of metastatic disease [87]. However, despite demonstration of effective MAPK inhibition, these MEK inhibitors have not shown to improve patient outcomes, neither in progression-free nor in overall survival rates [82].

6.2 HER2 inhibitors

HER2 is a member of the EGFR pathway. Ligand-bound receptors heterodimerize with HER2 proteins, which activates this pathway [88]. HER2 overexpression is commonly implicated in malignancy, including breast, gastric, lung, and colorectal cancers. This overexpression is caused by gene amplification, allowing for this pathway to proceed irrespective of the aforementioned ligand-bound receptors [89].

HER2 overexpression or amplification represents a small proportion of CRC cases, estimated between 1% and 3% depending on tumor stage [82, 90]. And, even in this small proportion of cases, HER2-targeted agents were shown to have low response rate when used as a monotherapy, or when used in combination with only chemotherapy [82]. Yet, there are more promising developments in low-toxicity, HER2-based, dual-targeted therapies that portend high disease control. One combination therapy—trastuzumab (a HER2 inhibitor) and lapatinib (an antineoplastic agents and tyrosine kinase inhibitor)—was studied in the recent HERACLES trials demonstrating this potential [91].

6.3 BRAF inhibitors

BRAF inhibitors target the BRAF gene, which is, too, involved in the RAS-MAPK signaling pathway [92]. In cases of CRC, patients routinely undergo molecular testing of RAS and BRAF genes, and those with mutations in the latter are known to have poorer prognoses [93]. This subset represents an estimated 12% of cases [94]. And, nearly one-third of this subset harbors microsatellite instability, which represents a target for BRAF-based therapy [95].

Similar to HER2 inhibitors, a BRAF-based, dual-targeted agent portends improved outcomes compared to BRAF inhibitor monotherapy. Combination therapies include those alongside anti-EGFR agents or MEK inhibitors [93]. This therapy most typically includes a combination of encorafenib (BRAF inhibitor) and cetuximab (EGF antibody) after first-line bevacizumab/chemotherapy [96]. This regimen was developed and demonstrated effective in the series of BEACON trials exploring BRAF V600E-mutated metastatic colorectal cancer [97].

7. Conclusion

Colorectal cancer is a highly pervasive diagnosis within the United States, both in terms of incidence of disease, as well as morbidity and mortality of patients upon diagnosis. It is the fourth highest cancer in incidence and second highest rate of cancer-related mortality [3].

Therefore, there is also ample research and development dedicated to curating colorectal cancer therapies: in bolstering current therapies, in expanding novel immunotherapies and targeted therapies, in combining agents with longstanding chemo- and radiation therapies, and in promoting and prioritizing new vaccines targeted against colorectal cancer subtypes.

These current therapies are typically based on cancer staging, ranging from simple surgical resection and monitoring for early stage colorectal cancers [29], to chemotherapy and biologic agents for advanced, metastatic disease [32, 33]. When appropriate, the current approach involves treating with chemotherapy with or without radiation therapy, followed by surgical intervention, and finally completed with adjuvant chemotherapy. These surgical procedures are typically performed under minimally invasive approaches, but again are limited in the case of even locally spread disease.

More novel treatment strategies, on the other hand, include targeted therapies, immunotherapies, vaccines, and cellular therapies, which are used in both isolation and combination with other agents discussed, and particularly against advanced, metastatic disease.

The most common genes targeted in such directed therapies include those related to mitogen-activated protein kinase, human epidermal growth factor receptor two, and BRAF genes [83]. Immunotherapies, on the other hand, typically consist of immune checkpoint inhibitors and are particularly effective in colorectal cancers involving microsatellite instability-high or mismatch-repair-deficient tumors [17].

Approved agents included pembrolizumab (shown to have 7% complete response rate [19], and now considered first-line therapy for metastatic colorectal cancers with microsatellite instability-high or mismatch-repair-deficient tumors [20]), as well as nivolumab and ipilimumab (undergoing further study but with promising early applications in similar metastatic cases [21]). These agents are also being investigated in combination with other longstanding therapies, including alongside chemotherapy and VEGF inhibitors. This therapeutic approach is therefore a promising area of active research as it applies to colorectal cancer.

Vaccines are another largely untapped area of future research as it pertains to colorectal cancer subtypes. These approaches would theoretically target tumor-associated antigens, tumor proteins, and tumor-specific antigens.

Finally, within the realm of these novel therapies, cell-directed therapies are an important area of evolving research. These agents are immune cells that are genetically modified to specifically target tumor cell types.

These agents are in constant evolution, both in expanding their individual effects, as well as in their efficacy in conjunction with the abovementioned current therapies.

Future research is needed to better assess the rising incidence of early-onset colorectal cancer, as well as the implications of the current lines of therapy against this evolving landscape of the population of colorectal cancer patients [9]. Preliminary data suggests that these cases are related to both hereditary causes (16% of patients with germline mutations) and lifestyle factors (diet, exercise, metabolic syndrome, alcohol consumption) [11, 98]. Yet, further exploration is necessary to further elucidate out these and other factors that may be contributing to these changing cancer incidence.

Author details

Muriel Battaglia[1†], Susan L. Feldt[1†], Marcus Marable[1†] and Ardaman Shergill[2*]

1 Department of Medicine, University of Chicago, USA

2 Section of Hematology/Oncology, Department of Medicine, University of Chicago, USA

*Address all correspondence to: ashergill@bsd.uchicago.edu

† First author.

References

[1] SEER. Cancer of the Colon and Rectum—Cancer Stat Facts. Available from: https://seer.cancer.gov/statfacts/html/colorect.html [Accessed: March 6, 2024]

[2] Sung H, Ferlay J, Siegel RL, Laversanne M, Soerjomataram I, Jemal A, et al. Global cancer statistics 2020: GLOBOCAN estimates of incidence and mortality worldwide for 36 cancers in 185 countries. CA: A Cancer Journal for Clinicians. 2021;**71**(3):209-249. DOI: 10.3322/caac.21660

[3] Siegel RL, Miller KD, Sauer AG, Fedewa SA, Butterly LF, Anderson JC, et al. Colorectal cancer statistics, 2020. CA: A Cancer Journal for Clinicians. 2020;**70**(3):145-164. DOI: 10.3322/caac.21601

[4] Brenner H, Stock C, Hoffmeister M. Effect of screening sigmoidoscopy and screening colonoscopy on colorectal cancer incidence and mortality: Systematic review and meta-analysis of randomised controlled trials and observational studies. British Medical Journal (Clinical Research Ed.). 2014;**348**:g2467. DOI: 10.1136/bmj.g2467

[5] Siegel RL, Miller KD, Wagle NS, Jemal A. Cancer statistics, 2023. CA: A Cancer Journal for Clinicians. 2023;**73**(1):17-48. DOI: 10.3322/caac.21763

[6] Van Cutsem E, Cervantes A, Adam R, Sobrero A, Van Krieken JH, Aderka D, et al. ESMO consensus guidelines for the management of patients with metastatic colorectal cancer. Annals of Oncology. 2016;**27**(8):1386-1422. DOI: 10.1093/annonc/mdw235

[7] Patel SG, Karlitz JJ, Yen T, Lieu CH, Boland RC. The rising tide of early-onset colorectal cancer: A comprehensive review of epidemiology, clinical features, biology, risk factors, prevention, and early detection. The Lancet Gastroenterology & Hepatology. 2022;7(3):262-274. Available from: https://www.thelancet.com/journals/langas/article/PIIS2468-1253(21)00426-X/abstract. [Accessed: March 6, 2024]

[8] Rex DK, Richard Boland C, Dominitz JA, Giardiello FM, Johnson DA, Kaltenbach T, et al. Colorectal cancer screening: Recommendations for physicians and patients from the U.S. multi-society task force on colorectal cancer. Gastroenterology. 2017;**153**(1):307-323. DOI: 10.1053/j.gastro.2017.05.013

[9] Bailey CE, Chung-Yuan H, Nancy You Y, Bednarski BK, Rodriguez-Bigas MA, Skibber JM, et al. Increasing disparities in the age-related incidences of colon and rectal cancers in the United States, 1975-2010. JAMA Surgery. 2015;**150**(1):17-22. DOI: 10.1001/jamasurg.2014.1756

[10] Siegel RL, Torre LA, Soerjomataram I, Hayes RB, Bray F, Weber TK, et al. Global patterns and trends in colorectal cancer incidence in young adults. Gut. **68**(12):2179-2185. Available from: https://gut.bmj.com/content/68/12/2179. [Accessed: March 6, 2024]

[11] Pearlman R, Frankel WL, Swanson B, Zhao W, Yilmaz A, Miller K, et al. Prevalence and spectrum of germline cancer susceptibility gene mutations among patients with early-onset colorectal cancer. JAMA Oncology. 2017;**3**(4):464-471. DOI: 10.1001/jamaoncol.2016.5194

[12] Center for Drug Evaluation and Research. FDA Approves Trifluridine

and Tipiracil with Bevacizumab for Previously Treated Metastatic Colorectal Cancer. Silver Spring, MD, USA: FDA; 2023. Available from: https://www.fda.gov/drugs/drug-approvals-and-databases/fda-approves-trifluridine-and-tipiracil-bevacizumab-previously-treated-metastatic-colorectal-cancer

[13] Ribas A, Wolchok JD. Cancer immunotherapy using checkpoint blockade. Science. 2018;**359**(6382):1350-1355. DOI: 10.1126/science.aar4060

[14] Ribas A, Hamid O, Adil Daud F, Hodi S, Wolchok JD, Kefford R, et al. Association of pembrolizumab with tumor response and survival among patients with advanced melanoma. JAMA. 2016;**315**(15):1600-1609. DOI: 10.1001/jama.2016.4059

[15] Garon EB, Rizvi NA, Hui R, Leighl N, Balmanoukian AS, Eder JP, et al. Pembrolizumab for the treatment of non–small-cell lung cancer. New England Journal of Medicine. 2015;**372**(21):2018-2028. DOI: 10.1056/NEJMoa1501824

[16] Mulet-Margalef N, Linares J, Badia-Ramentol J, Jimeno M, Monte CS, Mozo JLM, et al. Challenges and therapeutic opportunities in the dMMR/MSI-H colorectal cancer landscape. Cancers. 2023;**15**(4):1022. DOI: 10.3390/cancers15041022

[17] Sinicrope F, Foster NR, Sargent DJ, Gallinger S, Benatti P, Marsoni S, et al. DNA mismatch repair status and site of tumor recurrence in stage II and III colon cancers treated in 5-fluorouracil-based adjuvant therapy trials. Journal of Clinical Oncology. 2010;**28**(Suppl. 15): 3519-3519. DOI: 10.1200/jco.2010.28.15_suppl.3519

[18] Le DT, Uram JN, Wang H, Bartlett BR, Kemberling H, Eyring AD, et al. PD-1 blockade in tumors with mismatch-repair deficiency. New England Journal of Medicine. 2015;**372**(26):2509-2520. DOI: 10.1056/NEJMoa1500596

[19] Marcus L, Lemery SJ, Keegan P, Pazdur R. FDA approval summary: Pembrolizumab for the treatment of microsatellite instability-high solid tumors. Clinical Cancer Research. 2019;**25**(13):3753-3758. DOI: 10.1158/1078-0432.CCR-18-4070

[20] André T, Shiu K-K, Kim TW, Jensen BV, Jensen LH, Punt C, et al. Pembrolizumab in microsatellite-instability–high advanced colorectal cancer. New England Journal of Medicine. 2020;**383**(23):2207-2218. DOI: 10.1056/NEJMoa2017699

[21] Lenz H-J, Van Cutsem E, Limon ML, Wong KYM, Hendlisz A, Aglietta M, et al. First-line nivolumab plus low-dose ipilimumab for microsatellite instability-high/mismatch repair-deficient metastatic colorectal cancer: The Phase II CheckMate 142 Study. Journal of Clinical Oncology. 2022;**40**(2):161-170. DOI: 10.1200/JCO.21.01015

[22] Lau D, Kalaitzaki E, Church DN, Pandha H, Tomlinson I, Annels N, et al. Rationale and design of the POLEM trial: Avelumab plus fluoropyrimidine-based chemotherapy as adjuvant treatment for stage III mismatch repair deficient or POLE exonuclease domain mutant colon cancer: A Phase III Randomised Study. ESMO Open. 2020;**5**(1):e000638. DOI: 10.1136/esmoopen-2019-000638

[23] Sinicrope FA, Fang-Shu O, Zemla T, Nixon AB, Mody K, Levasseur A, et al. Randomized trial of standard chemotherapy alone or combined with atezolizumab as adjuvant therapy for patients with stage III colon cancer and deficient mismatch repair (ATOMIC, Alliance A021502). Journal of Clinical

Oncology. 2019;**37**(Suppl. 15):e15169. DOI: 10.1200/JCO.2019.37.15_suppl.e15169

[24] Herting CJ, Farren MR, Tong Y, Liu Z, O'Neil B, Bekaii-Saab T, et al. A multi-center, single arm, phase Ib study of pembrolizumab (MK-3475) in combination with chemotherapy for patients with advanced colorectal cancer: HCRN GI14-186. Cancer Immunology, Immunotherapy: CII. 2021;**70**(11):3337-3348. DOI: 10.1007/s00262-021-02986-5

[25] Fukuoka S, Hara H, Takahashi N, Kojima T, Kawazoe A, Asayama M, et al. Regorafenib plus nivolumab in patients with advanced gastric or colorectal cancer: An open-label, dose-escalation, and dose-expansion phase Ib trial (REGONIVO, EPOC1603). Journal of Clinical Oncology. 2020;**38**(18):2053-2061. DOI: 10.1200/JCO.19.03296

[26] El-Khoueiry AB, Fakih M, Gordon MS, Tsimberidou AM, Bullock AJ, Wilky BA, et al. Results from a phase 1a/1b study of botensilimab (BOT), a novel innate/adaptive immune activator, plus balstilimab (BAL; anti-PD-1 antibody) in metastatic heavily pretreated microsatellite stable colorectal cancer (MSS CRC). Journal of Clinical Oncology. 2023;**41**(Suppl. 4):LBA8. DOI: 10.1200/JCO.2023.41.4_suppl.LBA8

[27] Kasi PM, Hidalgo M, Jafari MD, Yeo H, Lowenfeld L, Khan U, et al. Neoadjuvant botensilimab plus balstilimab response pattern in locally advanced mismatch repair proficient colorectal cancer. Oncogene. 2023;**42**(44):3252-3259. DOI: 10.1038/s41388-023-02835-y

[28] Amin MB, Greene FL, Edge SB, Compton CC, Gershenwald JE, Brookland RK, et al. The eighth edition AJCC cancer staging manual: Continuing to build a bridge from a population-based to a more 'personalized' approach to cancer staging. CA: A Cancer Journal for Clinicians. 2017;**67**(2):93-99. DOI: 10.3322/caac.21388

[29] Nash GM, Weiser MR, Guillem JG, Temple LK, Shia J, Mithat Gonen W, et al. Long-term survival after transanal excision of T1 rectal cancer. Diseases of the Colon & Rectum. 2009;**52**(4):577. DOI: 10.1007/DCR.0b013e3181a0adbd

[30] Ribic CM, Sargent DJ, Moore MJ, Thibodeau SN, French AJ, Goldberg RM, et al. Tumor microsatellite-instability status as a predictor of benefit from fluorouracil-based adjuvant chemotherapy for colon cancer. New England Journal of Medicine. 2003;**349**(3):247-257. DOI: 10.1056/NEJMoa022289

[31] Fleshman J, Branda ME, Sargent DJ, Boller AM, George VV, Abbas MA, et al. Disease-free survival and local recurrence for laparoscopic resection compared with open resection of stage II to III rectal cancer: Follow-up results of the ACOSOG Z6051 randomized controlled trial. Annals of Surgery. 2019;**269**(4):589. DOI: 10.1097/SLA.0000000000003002

[32] Fong Y, Cohen AM, Fortner JG, Enker WE, Turnbull AD, Coit DG, et al. Liver resection for colorectal metastases. Journal of Clinical Oncology. 1997;**15**(3):938-946. DOI: 10.1200/JCO.1997.15.3.938

[33] Inoue M, Kotake Y, Nakagawa K, Fujiwara K, Fukuhara K, Yasumitsu T. Surgery for pulmonary metastases from colorectal carcinoma. The Annals of Thoracic Surgery. 2000;**70**(2):380-383. DOI: 10.1016/S0003-4975(00)01417-X

[34] Keller DS, Berho M, Perez RO, Wexner SD, Chand M. The multidisciplinary management of rectal

cancer. Nature Reviews Gastroenterology & Hepatology. 2020;**17**(7):414-429. DOI: 10.1038/s41575-020-0275-y

[35] Fleshman J, Branda M, Sargent DJ, Boller AM, George V, Abbas M, et al. Effect of laparoscopic-assisted resection vs open resection of stage II or III rectal cancer on pathologic outcomes. JAMA. 2015;**314**(13):1346-1355. DOI: 10.1001/jama.2015.10529

[36] Vogel JD, Felder SI, Bhama AR, Hawkins AT, Langenfeld SJ, Shaffer VO, et al. The American society of colon and rectal surgeons clinical practice guidelines for the management of colon cancer. Diseases of the Colon & Rectum. 2022;**65**(2):148. DOI: 10.1097/DCR.0000000000002323

[37] Abdalla EK, Vauthey J-N, Ellis LM, Ellis V, Pollock R, Broglio KR, et al. Recurrence and outcomes following hepatic resection, radiofrequency ablation, and combined resection/ablation for colorectal liver metastases. Annals of Surgery. 2004;**239**(6):818-827. DOI: 10.1097/01.sla.0000128305.90650.71

[38] Sakamoto T, Tsubota N, Iwanaga K, Yuki T, Matsuoka H, Yoshimura M. Pulmonary resection for metastases from colorectal cancer. Chest. 2001;**119**(4):1069-1072. DOI: 10.1378/chest.119.4.1069

[39] Molla M, Fernandez-Plana J, Albiol S, Fondevila C, Vollmer I, Cases C, et al. Limited liver or lung colorectal cancer metastases. Systemic treatment, surgery, ablation or SBRT. Journal of Clinical Medicine. 2021;**10**(10):2131. DOI: 10.3390/jcm10102131

[40] Pisano M, Zorcolo L, Merli C, Cimbanassi S, Poiasina E et al. 2017 WSES guidelines on colon and rectal cancer emergencies: Obstruction and perforation. World Journal of Emergency Surgery. **13**:1-27. Available from: https://wjes.biomedcentral.com/articles/10.1186/s13017-018-0192-3. [Accessed: March 6, 2024]

[41] Martenson JA, Willett CG, Sargent DJ, Mailliard JA, Donohue JH, Gunderson LL, et al. Phase III study of adjuvant chemotherapy and radiation therapy compared with chemotherapy alone in the surgical adjuvant treatment of colon cancer: Results of intergroup protocol 0130. Journal of Clinical Oncology. 2004;**22**(16):3277-3283. DOI: 10.1200/JCO.2004.01.029

[42] Moertel CG, Fleming TR, Macdonald JS, Haller DG, Laurie JA, Tangen CM, et al. Intergroup study of fluorouracil plus levamisole as adjuvant therapy for stage II/dukes' B2 colon cancer. Journal of Clinical Oncology. 1995;**13**(12):2936-2943. DOI: 10.1200/JCO.1995.13.12.2936

[43] Lembersky BC, Samuel Wieand H, Petrelli NJ, O'Connell MJ, Colangelo LH, Smith RE, et al. Oral uracil and tegafur plus leucovorin compared with intravenous fluorouracil and leucovorin in stage II and III carcinoma of the colon: Results from National Surgical Adjuvant Breast and Bowel Project Protocol C-06. Journal of Clinical Oncology: Official Journal of the American Society of Clinical Oncology. 2006;**24**(13):2059-2064. DOI: 10.1200/JCO.2005.04.7498

[44] Twelves C, Wong A, Nowacki MP, Abt M, Burris H, Carrato A, et al. Capecitabine as adjuvant treatment for stage III colon cancer. New England Journal of Medicine. 2005;**352**(26):2696-2704. DOI: 10.1056/NEJMoa043116

[45] André T, Boni C, Mounedji-Boudiaf L, Navarro M, Tabernero J, Hickish T, et al. Oxaliplatin, fluorouracil, and leucovorin as adjuvant treatment

for colon cancer. New England Journal of Medicine. 2004;**350**(23):2343-2351. DOI: 10.1056/NEJMoa032709

[46] Akdeniz N, Kaplan MA, Uncu D, İnanç M, Kaya S, Dane F, et al. The comparison of FOLFOX regimens with different doses of 5-FU for the adjuvant treatment of colorectal cancer: A multicenter study. International Journal of Colorectal Disease. 2021;**36**(6):1311-1319. DOI: 10.1007/s00384-021-03888-9

[47] Saltz LB, Niedzwiecki D, Hollis D, Goldberg RM, Hantel A, Thomas JP, et al. Irinotecan plus fluorouracil/leucovorin (IFL) versus fluorouracil/leucovorin alone (FL) in stage III colon cancer (intergroup trial CALGB C89803). Journal of Clinical Oncology. 2004;**22**(Suppl. 14):3500-3500. DOI: 10.1200/jco.2004.22.90140.3500

[48] Ychou M, Raoul J-L, Douillard J-Y, Bugat R, Mineur L, Viret F, et al. A phase III randomized trial of LV5FU2+CPT-11 vs. LV5FU2 alone in adjuvant high risk colon cancer (FNCLCC Accord02/FFCD9802). Journal of Clinical Oncology. 2005;**23**(Suppl. 16):3502-3502. DOI: 10.1200/jco.2005.23.16_suppl.3502

[49] Gluzman A, Rubinov K, Mermershtain W, Man S, Ariad S, Lavrenkov K. Retrospective comparison of two different schedules of irinotecan, 5-fluorouracil and folinic acid in previously untreated patients with advanced colorectal carcinoma: A single institution experience. Journal of Chemotherapy. 2007;**19**(6):739-743. DOI: 10.1179/joc.2007.19.6.739

[50] Ducreux M et al. Capecitabine plus oxaliplatin (XELOX) versus 5-fluorouracil/leucovorin plus oxaliplatin (FOLFOX-6) as first-line treatment for metastatic colorectal cancer. International Journal of Cancer. 2011;**128**(3):682-690. Available from: https://onlinelibrary.wiley.com/doi/10.1002/ijc.25369 [Accessed: March 6, 2024]

[51] Rothenberg ML, Cox JV, Butts C, Navarro M, Bang Y-J, Goel R, et al. Capecitabine plus oxaliplatin (XELOX) versus 5-fluorouracil/folinic acid plus oxaliplatin (FOLFOX-4) as second-line therapy in metastatic colorectal cancer: A Randomized Phase III Noninferiority Study. Annals of Oncology. 2008;**19**(10):1720-1726. DOI: 10.1093/annonc/mdn370

[52] Khali KA, Musalm HS, Hassan MA, Mahmoud IA. Triplet (FOLFOXIRI) versus doublet (FOLFOX or FOLFIRI) regimen as first line treatment in metastatic colorectal carcinoma, a prospective phase II, randomized controlled trial. Asian Pacific Journal of Cancer Prevention: APJCP. 2022;**23**(10):3421-3429. DOI: 10.31557/APJCP.2022.23.10.3421

[53] Hurwitz H, Fehrenbacher L, Novotny W, Cartwright T, Hainsworth J, Heim W, et al. Bevacizumab plus irinotecan, fluorouracil, and leucovorin for metastatic colorectal cancer. New England Journal of Medicine. 2004;**350**(23):2335-2342. DOI: 10.1056/NEJMoa032691

[54] Saltz LB, Clarke S, Díaz-Rubio E, Scheithauer W, Figer A, Wong R, et al. Bevacizumab in combination with oxaliplatin-based chemotherapy as first-line therapy in metastatic colorectal cancer: A Randomized Phase III Study. Journal of Clinical Oncology. 2008;**26**(12):2013-2019. DOI: 10.1200/JCO.2007.14.9930

[55] Cremolini C, Antoniotti C, Stein A, Bendell J, Gruenberger T, Rossini D, et al. Individual patient data meta-analysis of FOLFOXIRI plus bevacizumab versus doublets plus bevacizumab as initial

therapy of unresectable metastatic colorectal cancer. Journal of Clinical Oncology: Official Journal of the American Society of Clinical Oncology. 2020;**38**:JCO2001225. DOI: 10.1200/JCO.20.01225

[56] Bahadoer RR, Dijkstra EA, van Etten B, Marijnen CAM, Putter H, Kranenbarg EM-K, et al. Short-course radiotherapy followed by chemotherapy before total mesorectal excision (TME) versus preoperative chemoradiotherapy, TME, and optional adjuvant chemotherapy in locally advanced rectal cancer (RAPIDO): A randomised, open-label, phase 3 trial. The Lancet Oncology. 2021;**22**(1):29-42. DOI: 10.1016/S1470-2045(20)30555-6

[57] de Gramont A, Figer A, Seymour M, Homerin M, Hmissi A, Cassidy J, et al. Leucovorin and fluorouracil with or without oxaliplatin as first-line treatment in advanced colorectal cancer. Journal of Clinical Oncology. 2023;**41**(33):5080-5089. DOI: 10.1200/JCO.22.02773

[58] Lin EH, Skibber J, Delcos M, Eng C, Christopher C, Brown T, et al. A phase II study of capecitabine and concomitant boost radiotherapy (XRT) in patients (pts) with locally advanced rectal cancer (LARC). Journal of Clinical Oncology. 2005;**23**(Suppl. 16):3593-3593. DOI: 10.1200/jco.2005.23.16_suppl.3593

[59] Fokas E, Schlenska-Lange A, Polat B, Klautke G, Grabenbauer GG, Fietkau R, et al. Chemoradiotherapy plus induction or consolidation chemotherapy as total neoadjuvant therapy for patients with locally advanced rectal cancer: Long-term results of the CAO/ARO/AIO-12 randomized clinical trial. JAMA Oncology. 2022;**8**(1):e215445. DOI: 10.1001/jamaoncol.2021.5445

[60] Conroy T, Etienne P, Rio E, Evesque L, Mesgouez-Nebout N, et al. Total neoadjuvant therapy with mFOLFIRINOX versus preoperative chemoradiation in patients with locally advanced rectal cancer: 7-year results of PRODIGE 23 phase III trial, a UNICANCER GI trial. Journal of Clinical Oncology. **41**(17). Available from: https://ascopubs.org/doi/abs/10.1200/JCO.2023.41.17_suppl.LBA3504. [Accessed: March 6, 2024]

[61] Van Cutsem E, Tabernero J, Lakomy R, Prenen H, Prausova J, et al. Addition of aflibercept to fluorouracil, leucovorin, and irinotecan improves survival in a phase III randomized trial in patients with metastatic colorectal cancer previously treated with an oxaliplatin-based regimen. Journal of Clinical Oncology. **30**(28):3499-3506. Available from: https://ascopubs.org/doi/10.1200/jco.2012.42.8201. [Accessed: March 6, 2024]

[62] Tabernero J, Cohn AL, Obermannova R, Bodoky G, Ciuleanu T, et al. RAISE: A randomized, double-blind, multicenter phase III study of irinotecan, folinic acid, and 5-fluorouracil (FOLFIRI) plus ramucirumab (RAM) or placebo (PBO) in patients (Pts) with metastatic colorectal carcinoma (CRC) progressive during or following first-line combination therapy with bevacizumab (Bev), oxaliplatin (Ox), and a fluoropyrimidine (Fp). Journal of Clinical Oncology. **33**(3). Available from: https://ascopubs.org/doi/abs/10.1200/jco.2015.33.3_suppl.512. [Accessed: March 6, 2024]

[63] Jonker DJ, O'Callaghan CJ, Karapetis CS, Zalcberg JR, Dongsheng T, Heather-Jane A, et al. Cetuximab for the treatment of colorectal cancer. New England Journal of Medicine. 2007;**357**(20):2040-2048. DOI: 10.1056/NEJMoa071834

[64] Watanabe J, Muro K, Shitara K, Yamazaki K, Shiozawa M, Ohori H, et al.

Panitumumab vs bevacizumab added to standard first-line chemotherapy and overall survival among patients with RAS wild-type, left-sided metastatic colorectal cancer: A randomized clinical trial. JAMA. 2023;**329**(15):1271-1282. DOI: 10.1001/jama.2023.4428

[65] Grothey A, Van Cutsem E, Sobrero A, Siena S, Falcone A, Ychou M, et al. Regorafenib monotherapy for previously treated metastatic colorectal cancer (CORRECT): An international, multicentre, randomised, placebo-controlled, phase 3 trial. The Lancet. 2013;**381**(9863):303-312. DOI: 10.1016/S0140-6736(12)61900-X

[66] Overman MJ, McDermott R, Leach JL, Lonardi S, Lenz H-J, Morse MA, et al. Nivolumab in patients with metastatic DNA mismatch repair-deficient or microsatellite instability-high colorectal cancer (CheckMate 142): An open-label, multicentre, phase 2 study. The Lancet Oncology. 2017;**18**(9):1182-1191. DOI: 10.1016/S1470-2045(17)30422-9

[67] Prager GW, Taieb J, Fakih M, Ciardiello F, Van Cutsem E, Elez E, et al. Trifluridine-tipiracil and bevacizumab in refractory metastatic colorectal cancer. The New England Journal of Medicine. 2023;**388**(18):1657-1667. DOI: 10.1056/NEJMoa2214963

[68] Dasari A, Lonardi S, Garcia-Carbonero R, Elez E, Yoshino T, Sobrero A, et al. Fruquintinib versus placebo in patients with refractory metastatic colorectal cancer (FRESCO-2): An international, multicentre, randomised, double-blind, phase 3 study. Lancet (London, England). 2023;**402**(10395):41-53. DOI: 10.1016/S0140-6736(23)00772-9

[69] Moingeon P. Cancer vaccines. Vaccine. 2001;**19**(11):1305-1326. DOI: 10.1016/S0264-410X(00)00372-8

[70] Kumai T, Yamaki H, Kono M, Hayashi R, Wakisaka R, Komatsuda H. Antitumor peptide-based vaccine in the limelight. Vaccine. 2022;**10**(1):70. DOI: 10.3390/vaccines10010070

[71] McCann N, O'Connor D, Lambe T, Pollard AJ. Viral vector vaccines. Current Opinion in Immunology. 2022;**77**:102210. DOI: 10.1016/j.coi.2022.102210

[72] Lin IYC, Van TTH, Smooker PM. Live-attenuated bacterial vectors: Tools for vaccine and therapeutic agent delivery. Vaccines. **3**(4):940-972. Available from: https://www.mdpi.com/2076-393X/3/4/940 [Accessed: March 6, 2024]

[73] Larocca C, Schlom J. Viral vector-based therapeutic cancer vaccines. Cancer Journal (Sudbury, Mass.). 2011;**17**(5):359-371. DOI: 10.1097/PPO.0b013e3182325e63

[74] Baban CK, Cronin M, O'Hanlon D, O'Sullivan GC, Tangney M. Bacteria as vectors for gene therapy of cancer. Bioengineered Bugs. 2010;**1**(6):385-394. DOI: 10.4161/bbug.1.6.13146

[75] Kumar R, Kumar P. Yeast-based vaccines: New perspective in vaccine development and application. FEMS Yeast Research. 2019;**19**(2):foz007. DOI: 10.1093/femsyr/foz007

[76] Santos PM, Butterfield LH. Dendritic cell-based cancer vaccines. Journal of Immunology (Baltimore, Md.: 1950). 2018;**200**(2):443-449. DOI: 10.4049/jimmunol.1701024

[77] Lin B, Likun D, Li H, Zhu X, Cui L, Li X. Tumor-infiltrating lymphocytes: Warriors fight against tumors powerfully. Biomedicine & Pharmacotherapy. 2020;**132**:110873. DOI: 10.1016/j.biopha.2020.110873

[78] Chu J, Gao F, Yan M, Zhao S, Yan Z, Shi B, et al. Natural killer cells:

A promising immunotherapy for cancer. Journal of Translational Medicine. 2022;**20**(1):240. DOI: 10.1186/s12967-022-03437-0

[79] Meng Y, Zhifu Y, Yefeng W, Tianzhao D, Chen S, Meng F, et al. Cell-based immunotherapy with cytokine-induced killer (CIK) cells: From preparation and testing to clinical application. Human Vaccines & Immunotherapeutics. 2017;**13**(6):1379-1387. DOI: 10.1080/21645515.2017.1285987

[80] Chohan KL, Siegler EL, Kenderian SS. CAR-T cell therapy: The efficacy and toxicity balance. Current Hematologic Malignancy Reports. 2023;**18**(2):9-18. DOI: 10.1007/s11899-023-00687-7

[81] Sundberg EJ, Deng L, Mariuzza RA. TCR recognition of peptide/MHC class II complexes and superantigens. Seminars in Immunology. The Structure and Function of Antigen Receptors. 2007;**19**(4):262-271. DOI: 10.1016/j.smim.2007.04.006

[82] Xie Y-H, Chen Y-X, Fang J-Y. Comprehensive review of targeted therapy for colorectal cancer. Signal Transduction and Targeted Therapy. 2020;**5**:22. DOI: 10.1038/s41392-020-0116-z

[83] Sakata S, Larson DW. Targeted therapy for colorectal cancer. Surgical Oncology Clinics. 2022;**31**(2):255-264. DOI: 10.1016/j.soc.2021.11.006

[84] Pancione M, Giordano G, Parcesepe P, Cerulo L, Coppola L, Del Curatolo A, et al. Emerging insight into MAPK inhibitors and immunotherapy in colorectal cancer. Current Medicinal Chemistry. 2017;**24**(14):1383-1402

[85] Fang JY, Richardson BC. The MAPK signalling pathways and colorectal cancer. The Lancet Oncology. 2005;**6**(5):322-327. DOI: 10.1016/S1470-2045(05)70168-6

[86] Ellis LM, Ghosh S, Fan F, Bhattacharya R, Powell R, Park YS, et al. 35P enhancing efficacy of the MEK inhibitor trametinib in KRAS-mutated colorectal cancer cells. ESMO Open. 2023;**8**(1). DOI: 10.1016/j.esmoop.2023.101681

[87] Subbiah V, Baik C, Kirkwood JM. Clinical development of BRAF plus MEK inhibitor combinations. Trends in Cancer. 2020;**6**(9):797-810. DOI: 10.1016/j.trecan.2020.05.009

[88] Hynes NE, Lane HA. ERBB receptors and cancer: The complexity of targeted inhibitors. Nature Reviews Cancer. 2005;**5**(5):341-354. DOI: 10.1038/nrc1609

[89] Siena S, Sartore-Bianchi A, Marsoni S, Hurwitz HI, McCall SJ, Penault-Llorca F, et al. Targeting the human epidermal growth factor receptor 2 (HER2) oncogene in colorectal cancer. Annals of Oncology. 2018;**29**(5):1108-1119. DOI: 10.1093/annonc/mdy100

[90] Richman SD, Southward K, Chambers P, Cross D, Barrett J, Hemmings G, et al. HER2 overexpression and amplification as a potential therapeutic target in colorectal cancer: Analysis of 3256 patients enrolled in the QUASAR, FOCUS and PICCOLO colorectal cancer trials. The Journal of Pathology. 2016;**238**(4):562-570. DOI: 10.1002/path.4679

[91] Sartore-Bianchi A, Lonardi S, Martino C, Fenocchio E, Tosi F, Ghezzi S, et al. Pertuzumab and trastuzumab emtansine in patients with HER2-amplified metastatic colorectal cancer: The phase II HERACLES-B trial. ESMO Open. 2020;**5**(5):1-8. DOI: 10.1136/esmoopen-2020-000911

[92] Proietti I, Skroza N, Michelini S, Mambrin A, Balduzzi V, Bernardini N, et al. BRAF inhibitors: Molecular targeting and immunomodulatory actions. Cancers. 2020;**12**(7):1823. DOI: 10.3390/cancers12071823

[93] Ducreux M, Chamseddine A, Laurent-Puig P, Smolenschi C, Hollebecque A, Dartigues P, et al. Molecular targeted therapy of BRAF-mutant colorectal cancer. Therapeutic Advances in Medical Oncology. 2019;**11**:1758835919856494. DOI: 10.1177/1758835919856494

[94] Ros J, Rodríguez-Castells M, Saoudi N, Baraibar I, Salva F, Tabernero J, et al. Treatment of BRAF-V600E mutant metastatic colorectal cancer: New insights and biomarkers. Expert Review of Anticancer Therapy. 2023;**23**(8):797-806. DOI: 10.1080/14737140.2023.2236794

[95] Tabernero J, Ros J, Élez E. The evolving treatment landscape in BRAF-V600E–mutated metastatic colorectal cancer. American Society of Clinical Oncology Educational Book. 2022;**42**:254-263. DOI: 10.1200/EDBK_349561

[96] Ciombor KK, Strickler JH, Bekaii-Saab TS, Yaeger R. BRAF-mutated advanced colorectal cancer: A rapidly changing therapeutic landscape. Journal of Clinical Oncology. 2022;**40**(24):2706-2715. DOI: 10.1200/JCO.21.02541

[97] Kopetz S, Grothey A, Yaeger R, Van Cutsem E, Desai J, Yoshino T, et al. Encorafenib, binimetinib, and cetuximab in BRAF V600E–mutated colorectal cancer. New England Journal of Medicine. 2019;**381**(17):1632-1643. DOI: 10.1056/NEJMoa1908075

[98] Patel SG, Karlitz JJ, Yen T, Lieu CH, Richard Boland C. The rising tide of early-onset colorectal cancer: A comprehensive review of epidemiology, clinical features, biology, risk factors, prevention, and early detection. The Lancet Gastroenterology & Hepatology. 2022;**7**(3):262-274. DOI: 10.1016/S2468-1253(21)00426-X

Chapter 5

Treatment of Metastatic Colorectal Cancer: Beyond Progression

Ali Kaan Güren and Osman Köstek

Abstract

Metastatic colorectal cancer is a major health problem, accounting for 8.1% of US cancer cases. Although 5-FU-oxaliplatin-irinotecan-based chemotherapy combination regimens and targeted therapies have increased 5-year survival rates to around 13%. The still low rate of this rate increases the demand for new treatment options. Advances in the discovery of tumor biology have made it possible to better define the subtypes and resistance mechanisms of metastatic colorectal cancer. In this regard, personalized treatment strategies are becoming increasingly important in the treatment of advanced stages of metastatic colorectal cancer. New therapeutic options, immune checkpoint inhibitors, monoclonal antibodies against various targets, and multitargeted tyrosine kinase inhibitors are available in the treatment of later lines of metastatic colorectal cancer. The treatment strategy is based on patients' performance status, residual toxicity, and especially molecular profile.

Keywords: treatment, metastatic colorectal cancer, beyond progression, immunotherapy, rechallenge, monoclonal antibody

1. Introduction

Metastatic colorectal cancer (mCRC) is the third most common cause of newly diagnosed cancer and the second most common cause of cancer-related death in both sexes [1]. Approximately, 8.1% of newly diagnosed cancer cases in the United States are colorectal cancers. At the time of diagnosis, approximately, 21% of patients are diagnosed in the metastatic stage. As systemic treatment options, 5 fluorouracil (5-FU)-based chemotherapy combination regimens with monoclonal antibodies, multitargeted kinase inhibitors alone, and immunotherapy agents are important treatment arguments. With these treatment options, 5-year survival rates in patients with metastatic colorectal cancer have improved significantly, reaching approximately 13% [2]. In addition, according to the surveillance epidemiology and end results (SEER) medicare database analysis for mCRC, the increase in treatment lines correlates with an increase in overall survival times (**Figure 1**) [3]. In other words, in unresectable mCRC patients who exhausted the first two lines of treatment options, overall survival (OS) durations of 23–24 months are known to increase with the drugs used after beyond progression, with a significant additional contribution to overall OS durations. In addition, after the first two treatment lines, approximately, 63.3% of patients at baseline can reach to the third-line setting [4]. Designing the treatment

IntechOpen

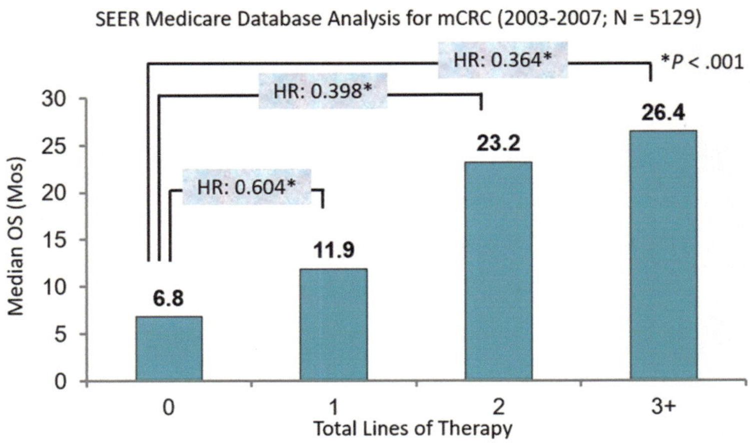

Figure 1.
Overall survival correlated with increased treatment lines.

regimen for patients who have progressed to the third-line setting should be acknowledged as the "art of science." Because the probability rate of clinical benefit with treatment in this patient group is approximately 35.2% [4]. In these patients, comorbidity and performance status, tumor burden, residual toxicity, and most importantly, the current molecular profile of the disease (biomarker analysis) should be considered at beyond progression. Moreover, an investigation into the genomic landscape of this ailment has allowed to therapeutic expansion, encompassing targeted therapies and immunotherapy. Given these considerations, treatment options can be divided into two groups: biomarker-driven therapy or non-biomarker-driven treatment pathways. In this section, treatment standards and especially current approaches will be mentioned, especially in terms of the standard treatment approach, which is limited especially after beyond progression, and an evaluation was made in terms of the current developments in terms of precision medicine.

2. Biomarker—driven treatment options

2.1 dMMR/MSI-H status

Mismatch repair deficient/high microsatellite instability (dMMR/MSI-H) status is recognized as a tumor-agnostic biomarker, demonstrating potential benefits from immunotherapy when identified across all solid cancers. In clinical studies, its prevalence has been reported to be approximately 4–5% in patients with metastatic colorectal cancer [5]. Deficiency in the protein products of the MSH2, PMS-2, MLH1, and MSH6 genes results in an inability to efficiently detect mismatched and unpaired bases, leading to the expression of abnormal proteins that can be recognized by the immune system as neoantigens. It is a poor prognostic marker before the era of immunotherapy and has been particularly associated with resistance to conventional 5-FU-based chemotherapy combinations. These patients may have both sporadic and familial dMMR. In patients with sporadic dMMR, tumor location is more likely to be a proximal colon, high grade, mucinous pathology, diploid, and closely associated with BRaf proto-oncogene (BRAF) V600E mutations. Approximately, one in four patients with dMMR present with familial Lynch syndrome. Sporadic dMMR tumors differ from familial dMMR-Lynch syndrome in terms of female gender, smoking, and younger age at diagnosis. Although individuals with Lynch syndrome typically receive a diagnosis at an age below 45, it is essential to consider the possibility of concurrent or subsequent extra-colonic tumors.

Patients with deficient mismatch repair (dMMR) status are eligible for immunotherapy in any line of therapy. In cases where these patients undergo chemotherapy in the initial two lines and experience disease progression, the subsequent line of therapy is appropriate for immunotherapy treatment. Checkpoint inhibitor treatment options encompass nivolumab ± ipilimumab, pembrolizumab, or dostarlimab-gxly (**Table 1**).

The KEYNOTE 164 study conducted a thorough investigation into the efficacy of pembrolizumab among patients diagnosed with mCRC characterized by MSH or dMMR. This patient cohort had undergone at least one series of standard therapy. KEYNOTE-164, a phase 2 study, enrolled a total of 124 participants. Cohort A was stratified based on patients who had undergone one or more sequential treatments, while cohort B was categorized into patients who had received two or more sequential treatments. The objective response rate was 33% (95% CI, 21–46%) for both cohort A and cohort B, and the median duration of response was not reached in either cohort. The median progression-free survival (PFS) was 2.3 months (95% CI, 2.1–8.1) for cohort A and 4.1 months (95% CI, 2.1–18.9) for cohort B. Median overall survival was 31.4 months (95% CI, 21.4 months to not reached) for cohort A and not reached (95% CI, 19.2 months to not reached) for cohort B. The rates of Grade 3–4 side effects were similar in the two groups [6]. The responses obtained with the use of pembrolizumab in MSI-H/dMMR CRC proved that the use of pembrolizumab is appropriate in patients with MSI-H/dMMR CRC, regardless of mutation status and the number of prior lines of therapy. It showed us that we should consider the option of immunotherapy in patients with MSI-H/dMMR CRC who have not received immunotherapy before.

The efficacy of nivolumab was investigated in the CheckMate-142 studies. A phase 2 cohort first published in 2017 investigated the efficacy of nivolumab in patients

Study	Phase	Agent	Line	Outcome
Keynote-164	Phase 2	Pembrolizumab	≥ 2 prior lines	ORR: 33% PFS: 2.3 mo OS: 31.4 mo
		Pembrolizumab	≥ 1 prior lines	ORR: 33% PFS: 4.1 mo OS: NR
Checkmate-142	Phase 2	Nivolumab	≥ 2 prior lines	ORR: 35.8% 1-year PFS: 50.4% 1-year OS: 73.4%
		Nivolumab+Ipilimumab	≥ 2 prior lines	ORR:65% (CR:13%) PFS: NR OS: NR
Garnet*	Phase 1	Dostarlimab	≥ 2 prior lines	ORR: 43.5% PFS: 8.4 mo OS: NR

**32.1% of study population was mCRC.*

Table 1.
ICIs in patients with chemotherapy-refractory mCRC.

with dMMR mCRC who had received at least one prior series of standard therapy. Nivolumab was administered IV at a dose of 3 mg/kg every 2 weeks. While complete response could not be achieved, partial response was achieved in 23 patients and stable disease in 28 patients. The objective response rate (ORR) for these patients was 31.1% (95% CI, 20.8–42.9), and 69% of patients achieved disease control for at least 3 months. 1-year PFS was 50% and OS was 73%. ORR was 28.6% in 21 patients with programmed death-ligand 1 (PDL-1) ≥1%, and ORR was 27.7% in 47 patients with PDL-1 < 1%. Grade 3–4 adverse events were observed in 20% patients [7]. These results in patients with dMMR mCRC showed that nivolumab alone had a positive effect on treatment response independent of tumor PD-L1 expression level.

Another cohort within CheckMate-142 investigated the efficacy of nivolumab plus ipilimumab in patients with dMMR mCRC who had received at least one prior series of therapy. In the study of 119 patients, 76% had received two or more series of standard therapy. Patients received nivolumab (3 mg/kg) plus ipilimumab (1 mg/kg) at 3-week intervals (four doses) followed by nivolumab (3 mg/kg) at 2-week intervals. ORR increased from 55% at 13.4 months to 65% at 50.9 months, and disease control rate was 81%. Complete response (CR) rate increased from 3% at 13.4 months to 13% at 50.9 months. Partial response (PR) was observed in 52% of patients, stable disease (SD) in 21%, and progressive disease (PD) in 12%. Adverse events occurred in 32% of patients, and 13% had to discontinue treatment due to adverse events [8]. These results demonstrated the long-term benefit of the combination of nivolumab and ipilimumab in treatment-refractory MSI-H/dMMR mCRC patients.

Dostarlimab is a humanized anti-PD-1 monoclonal antibody that acts by binding to the PD-1 receptor [9]. The efficacy of dostarlimab was first demonstrated in MSI-H metastatic or recurrent endometrial cancer [10]. Next, the efficacy of the GARNET study in the F cohort of non-endometrial solid tumors previously treated with dMMR was demonstrated. Of the 106 patients in this cohort, 69 were diagnosed with CRC. Patients received 500 mg dostarlimab Q3W for four cycles followed by 1000 mg Q6W until progression. The ORR in patients with mCRC was 36.2% (CI 25.0–48.7%) [11]. Based on the outcomes derived from this cohort, dostarlimab has emerged as a viable treatment option for patients with dMMR mCRC who have undergone previous therapeutic options.

Currently, with the dMMR test serving as the primary reflex test, immune checkpoint inhibitor options are employed as the initial treatment for patients in this group. In instances where patients experience progression following IO, they are transitioned to other therapeutic options rather than immunotherapy options.

2.2 Anti-HER-2 treatments

HER-2 (human epidermal growth factor receptor 2) is a transmembrane protein and a member of the human epidermal growth factor receptor family. It acquires oncogenic characteristics through amplification or overexpression, potentially leading to the development of various cancers. One of these cancers is colorectal cancer [12]. It is detected in approximately 2–6% of colorectal cancers [13]. Currently, for patients with chemorefractory HER2-positive and RAS wild-type mCRC, there is evidence supporting the utilization of a dual anti-HER2 regimen. Tucatinib plus trastuzumab regimen has received initial FDA approval for this specific clinical scenario [14]. Furthermore, a combined PFS of 6.2 months indicates that HER2-targeted treatment regimens are linked with a significant enhancement in survival outcomes within this population (**Table 2**) [15].

Study	Phase	Agent	Line	Outcome
MyPathway	Phase 2	Trastuzumab+Pertuzumab	≥ 2 prior lines	ORR: 38% PFS: 4.6 mo OS: 10.3 mo
HERACLES-A	Phase 2	Trastuzumab+Lapatinib	≥ 2 prior lines	ORR: 30% PFS: 5.3 mo OS: 11.5 mo
DESTINY-CRC01	Phase 2	Trastuzumab deruxtecan	≥ 2 prior lines	ORR: 45.3% PFS: 6.3 mo OS: 15.5 mo
MOUNTAINEER	Phase 2	Trastuzumab+Tucatinib	≥ 2 prior lines	ORR: 52.2% PFS: 8.1 mo OS: 18.7 mo

Table 2.
Anti-HER-2 treatment trials in patients with chemotherapy-refractory mCRC.

2.2.1 Trastuzumab and pertuzumab

The MyPathway, TAPUR, and TRIUMPH studies have investigated the effectiveness of the combination of trastuzumab and pertuzumab in patients with HER-2 positive mCRC who have undergone multiple lines of treatment. The MyPathway study is a multicenter, open-label, phase 2a, multiple-basket trial. A total of 57 patients were enrolled in the study, with one patient showing a complete response and 17 patients demonstrating partial responses. The ORR was determined to be 32% [95% CI 20–45]. The estimated median PFS was 2.9 months [95% CI 1.4–5.3], and the estimated median OS was 11.5 months [95% CI 7.7 – not estimable (NE)]. Additionally, four patients exhibited a response lasting longer than 12 months [13]. The TAPUR study was a phase 2 basket trial. A total of 28 patients with HER-2 amplification were enrolled in the study. In the ERBB2 amplification cohort, durable clinical benefit (DCB) and ORR were observed in 54 and 25% of patients, respectively. The median PFS and median OS (95% confidence interval) were 17.2 weeks [95% CI 11.1–27.4] and 60.0 weeks [95% CI 32.1 to 102.3], respectively [16]. The TRIUMPH study showed that these patients who had received multiple lines of treatment, the ORR was found to be 35%, and the median PFS was 4 months [17]. The most important observed side effects in these studies include anemia, lymphopenia, and left ventricular dysfunction.

2.2.2 Trastuzumab ve tucatinib

Tucatinib is an orally administered antitumoral agent that exerts its effects by reversibly inhibiting the HER-2 tyrosine kinase inhibition [18]. The MOUNTAINEER study was a global, phase 2 trial that included 117 patients with chemotherapy-resistant, HER2-positive, RAS wild-type, unresectable, or metastatic colorectal cancer. Tucatinib (300 mg orally twice daily) plus intravenous trastuzumab (initial loading dose of 8 mg/kg, followed by 6 mg/kg every 21 days) was administered. Patients were divided into three cohorts. In cohorts A and B, covering 84 patients, the combination of Tucatinib and trastuzumab was given, while in cohort C, tucatinib monotherapy was provided. In cohorts A and B, the overall response rate (ORR) was 38.1% [95% CI 27.7–49.3], with complete response in three patients and partial response in 29 patients. The median duration of response (DOR) was 12.4 months [95% CI 8.5–20.5]. Median progression-free survival (PFS) was 8.2 months [95% CI 4.2–10.3], and median overall survival (OS) was 24.1 months [95% CI 20.3–36.7]. Comparable positive outcomes were not achieved in cohort C [19]. The achievement of a median survival of 2 years in this metastatic patient group resistant to combination therapy can be considered promising for the future.

2.2.3 Trastuzumab deruxtecan (T-DXd)

Trastuzumab deruxtecan, an antibody-drug conjugate (ADC), is formed through the covalent binding of the humanized anti-HER2 IgG1 monoclonal antibody (mAb) and the topoisomerase 1 inhibitor deruxtecan [20]. The efficacy of Trastuzumab deruxtecan in patients with mCRC has been demonstrated through a phase 2 study, DESTINY-CRC01. The study included patients with HER2-positive mCRC who had received at least two prior lines of treatment. The patients were divided into two groups: Group A consisted of 53 patients with HER2-positive, immunohistochemistry (IHC) 3+ or IHC 2+/*in situ* hybridization (ISH)+, while Group B included 33 patients with IHC 2+/ISH- or IHC 1+. In Group A, the ORR was 45.3% [95% CI, 31.6–59.6], and the DCR was 83% [95% CI 70.2–91.9], with 24 partial responses and 20 patients showing stable disease. The median PFS and OS were 6.9 months [95% CI 4.1–8.7) and 15.5 months [95% CI 8.8–20.8], respectively. In Group B, the ORR was 0% [21]. This study not only demonstrated the efficacy of Trastuzumab deruxtecan but also highlighted the importance of considering Trastuzumab deruxtecan as an option, particularly in patients with IHC 3+ or IHC 2+/ISH+.

2.2.4 Trastuzumab ve lapatinib

Lapatinib, epidermal growth factor receptor (HER1/EGFR/ERBB1) and HER2/ERBB2 inhibition, is a dual-acting oral antitumoral agent [22]. HERACLES, a multicenter, open-label, and phase 2 trial, was conducted to assess the effectiveness of the combination of trastuzumab and lapatinib in patients with mCRC who are KRAS wild-type and HER2 positive. Patients received IV trastuzumab at a loading dose of 4 mg/kg, followed by maintenance doses of 2 mg/kg weekly, along with oral lapatinib at a dose of 1000 mg daily. Out of the 27 patients included in the study, eight achieved an objective response [%30, 95% CI 14–50]; one patient achieved CR [%4, 95% CI 3–11], and seven patients achieved PR [%26, 95% CI 9–43]. SD was observed in 12 patients [%44, 95% CI GA 25–63]. No serious drug-related side effects were detected. The study concluded that the combination of trastuzumab and lapatinib demonstrated antitumoral efficacy in HER2-positive mCRC patients resistant to treatment [23].

2.3 KRAS G12C inhibitors

The KRASG12C mutation is identified in 2–4% of mCRC. The presence of the KRASG12C mutation is associated with a poor response to chemotherapy and an unfavorable prognosis. Selective KRASG12C inhibitors, such as sotorasib and adagrasib, have demonstrated indications of antitumor activity in mCRC. Adagrasib and sotorasib are agents developed against the KRAS G12C mutation. They function by irreversibly binding to the cysteine protein of KRAS G12C, thereby blocking KRAS signaling. This interruption halts cell growth and induces apoptosis [24]. Initially investigated for the treatment of non-small cell lung cancer, the use of these agents has later come to the forefront in the treatment of mCRC patients.

Sotorasib monotherapy was initially investigated in a phase 1–2 basket study known as the CodeBreaK trial. In the phase 1 portion of the study, a disease control rate of 73.8% was achieved in 42 patients with mCRC. In the phase 2 portion, objective response was observed in 9.7% of the 62 patients [25]. Subsequently, in December 2023, the results of a phase 3 randomized study comparing the combination of *sotorasib and panitumumab* with standard treatments were published. In this study, there were 53 patients in the sotorasib 960 mg and panitumumab arm, 53 patients in the sotorasib 2400 mg and panitumumumab group, and 54 patients in the standard treatment arm receiving regorafenib or trifluridine-tipiracil. Although OS data was not mature, median PFS was 2.2 months [95% CI, 1.9–3.9] in the standard care group, median PFS was 5.6 months [95% CI, 4.2–6.3) in the 960 mg sotorasib-panitumumab group, and median PFS was 3.9 months (95% CI, 3.7–5.8) in the 240 mg sotorasib-panitumumab groups. Compared with the standard care group, the hazard ratio for disease progression or mortality was 0.49 [95% CI, 0.30 to 0.80; P = 0.006] in the 960 mg sotorasib-panitumumab group and 0.58 [95% CI, 0.36 to 0.93; P = 0.03] in the 240 mg sotorasib-panitumumab group [26]. Based on the findings of this study, it can be concluded that the combination of sotorasib and panitumumab yielded more favorable results compared to sotorasib monotherapy.

Adagrasib was investigated in the KRYSTAL-1 study, focusing on patients with mCRC after studies involving solid tumors [27]. Then, current study compared adagrasib monotherapy with the combination of adagrasib and cetuximab in previously treated mCRC patients. Adagrasib was administered orally at 600 mg twice daily. Among the 44 patients treated with adagrasib monotherapy, responses were observed in 19% of patients [95% CI, 8 to 33]. The median response duration was 4.3 months [95% CI, 2.3–8.3], and the median progression-free survival was 5.6 months [95% CI, 4.1–8.3]. In the combination therapy group (*Adagrasib plus cetuximab*), the response rate was 46% [95% CI, 28–66]. The median response duration was 7.6 months [95% CI, 5.7 to not estimable], and the median progression-free survival was 6.9 months [95% CI, 5.4 to 8.1] [28].

These studies showed that adagrasib and sotorasib, both as monotherapy and in combination, had a positive effect on survival in patients with mCRC with KRAS 12C mutation. Although monotherapies appeared safer in terms of side effect profile, they had a more modest effect in terms of efficacy. In combination with panitumumab and cetuximab, the effects on survival appear to be more significant. In this respect, the guidelines primarily recommend combination therapies.

2.4 Anti-NTRK fusion-positive targets

RK fusions are infrequent but can be targeted mutations found across various cancer types. NTRK gene fusion is less common in CRC compared to other mutations (0.2–1%) [29]. Genetic profiling of 2519 colonic and rectal tumors revealed an approximate prevalence of 0.7% for NTRK-positive CRC [30]. Additionally, NTRK-positive CRC tumors demonstrated very high tumor mutation burden (median 53 mut/MB), microsatellite instability-high (MSI-H, 76%), and an enrichment of concurrent POLE and POLD1 mutations. This information can be valuable in directing molecularly driven treatment strategies, including targeted therapy and immunotherapy, for NTRK-positive CRC patients. Screening for NTRK fusions is recommended for patients with dMMR/MSI-H or high tumor mutational burden (TMB) CRC [30].

Larotrectinib and entrectinib are pan-tropomyosin receptor kinase (TRK) inhibitors that target TRKA, TRKB, and TRKC. These TRKs are encoded by the NTRK genes. The intracellular activation of these kinases normally regulates cell growth and differentiation. However, fusion proteins resulting from DNA damage in NTRK genes lead to uncontrolled cell growth. Larotrectinib and entrectinib inhibit these TRKs, preventing uncontrolled cell growth and differentiation. Importantly, they exhibit these effects in a tumor-agnostic manner, demonstrating efficacy across various types of cancer [31]. Indeed, due to their tumor-agnostic efficacy in targeting NTRK gene fusions, both larotrectinib and entrectinib, have received approval from regulatory bodies, such as the FDA (Food and Drug Administration) and EMA (European Medicines Agency). This approval allows the use of these drugs across various cancer types where NTRK gene fusions are present [32]. In a pooled analysis encompassing 55 patients under investigation for the efficacy of larotrectinib, it was observed that four patients exhibited colorectal cancer. The overall response rate, as determined by independent assessment, was 75% (95% CI, 61–85). At the end of the first year, responses were sustained in 71% of cases, and 55% of patients remained free of progression. Larotrectinib was administered orally at a dosage of 100 mg twice daily, and it was well-tolerated in 93% of patients. Third or fourth-degree AEs occurred in 5% of the patient population [33]. While larotrectinib and entrectinib have gained approval for tumor-agnostic use in solid tumors with NTRK fusion, it is crucial to note that the studies conducted, thus far have included a limited number of patients with mCRC. Consequently, there is a substantial disparity in treatment responses, with larotrectinib showing a 75% response rate compared to entrectinib's 25%. Given this divergence, it is imperative to conduct studies with larger patient cohorts to better demonstrate the efficacy of these agents in metastatic colorectal cancer. This will contribute to a more comprehensive understanding of their safety and effectiveness in the context of mCRC.

2.5 RET inhibitors

RET (Rearranged during Transfection) is a proto-oncogene that codes for a transmembrane receptor possessing a tyrosine kinase domain. Various alterations, such as mutations or rearrangements, lead to the activation of the kinase function of the receptor [34, 35].

In colorectal cancer, gene rearrangements have been reported in less than 1% of cases. Among these cases, common gene fusions identified in primary CRC tumors include ALK, ROS1, RET, NTRK3, BRAF, and RSPO1. These gene fusions represent a novel paradigm of oncogenic addiction in CRC [36]. Notably, tumors harboring RET fusions are characterized by their location in the right colon, older age at diagnosis, wild-type RAS and BRAF, and predominantly microsatellite instability-high (MSI-H), possibly defining a distinct subtype of colorectal cancer [37]. From a therapeutic perspective, given the highly positive results reported in phase II and III clinical trials for thyroid and lung cancers, there is an expectation that other types of tumors with positive RET status could benefit from anti-RET drugs. However, due to the rarity of such cases, conducting specific clinical trials for each disease is not feasible. Consequently, data regarding the antitumor activity of these drugs are often derived from early trials, emphasizing the need for further research and exploration in a broader range of cancer types with positive RET status. Selpercatinib is a receptor tyrosine kinase (RET) inhibitor. It is approved for use as a tumor agnostic in patients with RET fusion [38]. However, studies showing efficacy in mCRC are limited. Only 10 of the patients included in the phase 1–2 basket study LIBRETTO-001 were diagnosed with CRC. These patients had received at least two series of treatments. The ORR in the CRC group was 20% [95% CI, 2.5–55.6]. No complete response was detected in patients with CRC. The median duration of response for the colon cancer subgroup was 9.4 months [95% CI, 5.6–13.3]. Selpercatinib was used orally at a dose of 160 mg twice daily without interruption in phase 2 of the study [39]. While the use of selpercatinib in solid tumors is approved as tumor-agnostic, the LIBRETTO-001 study revealed that CR could not be achieved in patients with mCRC, and only 20% of patients showed a partial response. This underscores the necessity for studies with larger patient populations, specifically including those with mCRC, to better demonstrate efficacy. Further research in this context is crucial for a comprehensive understanding of the drug's effectiveness in treating metastatic colorectal cancer.

2.6 Anti-EGFR inhibitors rechallenge or reintroduction

Monoclonal antibodies that target the epidermal growth factor receptor (EGFR), such as cetuximab or panitumumab, represent foundational elements in the therapeutic approach to advanced-stage CRC [40]. As CRC progresses to the second, third, or fourth line of treatment, the overall prognosis for patients tends to worsen, and the available treatment options become more constrained. Additionally, a growing proportion of mCRC patients become ineligible for further cytotoxic chemotherapy, either due to a decline in performance status, severe adverse effects from prior chemotherapy, or personal choices made by the patients. Consequently, depending on the response to initial cytotoxic and anti-EGFR-based therapy, the rechallenge or reintroduction to anti-EGFR treatment emerges as a promising approach in later lines of treatment [41]. The CRICKET study, a prospective single-arm trial designed as a proof of concept, aimed to evaluate the efficacy of rechallenging with cetuximab plus irinotecan as a third-line treatment for patients with RAS and BRAF wild-type mCRC. The study demonstrated that anti-EGFR re-exposure exhibited clinical activity in mCRC cases that had developed acquired resistance to anti-EGFR treatment [42]. Additionally, a single-arm phase II CAVE trial (cetuximab rechallenge plus avelumab) enrolled 77 mCRC patients, concluding that cetuximab plus avelumab are effective treatment strategies with manageable toxicity profiles [43]. Conversely, the prospective CHRONOS trial has recently shown that liquid biopsy-driven rechallenge strategies can be considered feasible, offering potential improvements in clinical management [44]. Another study from a pooled analysis of the TRIBE and TRIBE2 studies investigated the efficacy of third and later-line treatments in subgroups of the study. This study included 1187 mCRC patients. After second progression, 53% of patients were able to receive treatment. In the subgroup analysis of patients with wild-type KRAS, NRAS, and BRAF, the administration of cetuximab or panitumumab as a third-line treatment resulted in a prolonged progression-free survival (PFS) compared to alternative treatments (6.4 vs. 3.9 months, $p = 0.02$). This finding suggests a potential benefit of using cetuximab or panitumumab in this specific patient subgroup [45]. Upon analysis of data from the CHRONOS, CRICKET, and TRIBE trials, it was observed that patients had undergone chemotherapy ± bevacizumab for a minimum of 4 months or longer in either the second series or in the previous series. This extended exposure to chemotherapy and bevacizumab may contribute to a reduction in the tumor population, potentially diminishing the presence of anti-EGFR resistance, thereby enhancing the efficacy of rechallenge with cetuximab or panitumumab in this patient group. Notably, the CHRONOS study demonstrated that the clearance of the RAS mutant allele, as determined by liquid biopsy, was similarly achieved within a 4-month as well [44]. Hence, it is noteworthy that within this patient population, a disease control rate of 63% was achieved, and there was evidence of prolongation in PFS [42, 44, 45]. Despite promising efficacy observed in prospective studies, there is a need for phase 3 trials conducted on a larger population to further validate these findings. Large-scale and well-designed phase 3 studies will provide more robust evidence regarding the effectiveness and safety of the rechallenge strategies in the treatment of metastatic colorectal cancer.

2.7 BRAF/MEK inhibitors

BRAF V600E mutation is observed in about 5–10% in patients with metastatic colorectal cancer, and this rate was found to be 9% in a meta-analysis of 6391 patients [46]. The efficacy of agents, such as encorafenib and vemurafenib, which are utilized in the treatment of other cancers, has been investigated in the management of metastatic colorectal cancer.

2.7.1 Vemurafenib

Vemurafenib is a competitive kinase inhibitor that acts against V600E mutated BRAF [47]. Its efficacy in the treatment of mCRC was demonstrated in the SWOG S1406 study, a randomized, phase 2 trial. The study included 106 patients with mCRC who had received at least 1 prior series of treatment. Patients were divided into two groups: irinotecan and cetuximab with or without vemurafenib (960 mg PO twice daily). Median PFS was 4.2 and 2.0 months in the vemurafenib and control arms, respectively. PFS was significantly longer in the vemurafenib arm [95% CI, 0.32–0.76, P = 0.001]. OS was not significantly different between the two arms [(HR, 0.77, 95% CI), 0.50–1.18, P = 0.23]. Response rate and disease control rate were 17% and 65% in the vemurafenib arm compared to 4% and 21% in the control arm [48]. The response rate and PFS duration demonstrated that the combination of vemurafenib with irinotecan and cetuximab is an option for patients with BRAF V600E mutant mCRC who have received multiple lines of therapy.

2.7.2 Encorafenib and cetuximab or panitumumab and/or binimetinib

Encorafenib is a small molecule BRAF inhibitor that targets enzymes in the MAPK signaling pathway [49]. Binimetinib is a potent and selective inhibitor of MEK (Mitogen-Activated Protein Kinase Kinase), and it is administered orally. MEK is a central kinase in the MAPK (Mitogen-Activated Protein Kinase) pathway, which plays a crucial role in promoting tumor growth [50]. The efficacy of the combination of encorafenib and cetuximab or panitumumumab in patients with mCRC was demonstrated in a phase 3 open-label study involving 665 patients. The study included patients with BRAF V600E mutated metastatic colorectal cancer whose disease progressed after one or two standard regimens. Patients were divided into three groups such as encorafenib, binimetinib, and cetuximab (triple therapy group), encorafenib and cetuximab (dual therapy group), and cetuximab and irinotecan or cetuximab and FOLFIRI (folinic acid, fluorouracil and irinotecan) (control group) in a 1:1:1 ratio. The median overall survival was 9.0 months in the triple therapy group and 5.4 months in the control group [HR 0.52; 95%CI, 0.39 to 0.70; P < 0.001]. The response rate was 26% [95% CI, 18–35] in the triple therapy group and 2% [95% CI, 0–7, P < 0.001] in the control group. The median overall survival in the dual treatment group was 8.4 months [HR vs. control, 0.60; 95% CI, 0.45 to 0.79; P < 0.001]. The response rate in the dual treatment group was 22% [95% CI, 14–33]. Grade 3 or higher adverse events occurred in 58% of patients in the triple treatment group, 50% in the dual treatment group, and 61% in the control group [51]. Adverse events were seen in more than 50%, but less frequently than in the standard arm. The combination of encorafenib and cetuximab, in particular the combination of encorafenib, cetuximab, and binimetinib, resulted in significantly longer overall survival and a higher response rate compared to standard therapy in previously treated patients with BRAF V600E mutation. This strengthens clinicians' hand for the future as an important weapon in mCRC patients with BRAF V600E mutation.

2.8 Tumor mutation burden or POLE mutations

Tumor mutational burden (TMB) quantifies the cumulative somatic coding mutations within a specific coding region of the tumor genome and is assessable through Next-generation sequencing (NGS) techniques. Extensive research has identified TMB as a potential biomarker indicative of immunotherapy response. Pembrolizumab has received FDA approval for patients with unresectable or metastatic solid tumors exhibiting high TMB (TMB-H), defined as 10 or more mutations/megabase by an FDA-approved test, who have progressed post-prior treatment with no satisfactory alternative options. The approval stems from the phase 2 study, KEYNOTE-158, involving patients with advanced solid tumors. In this study, those with TMB-H tumors treated with pembrolizumab demonstrated an ORR of 29%, contrasting with 6% in non-TMB-H tumors. A report from the phase II TAPUR basket study, focusing on 27 patients with TMB-H advanced CRC treated with pembrolizumab, noted one partial response and seven cases with stable disease for at least 16 weeks, resulting in a disease control rate of 28% and an ORR of 4%. Another TAPUR study abstract, covering 12 patients with TMB-H advanced CRC treated with nivolumab plus ipilimumab, concluded that this combination therapy lacks sufficient clinical activity in microsatellite stable, TMB-H CRC [52–54]. Although TMB-H demonstrated therapeutic significance in the KEYNOTE 158 study, some studies also showed that a TMB-H cutoff value of ≥10 for patients with MSS CRC was not associated with clinically meaningful response to immunotherapy.

Patients with colorectal cancer harboring POLE mutations exhibit distinctive clinical characteristics, including a younger age at diagnosis, a higher proportion of males compared to females, diagnosis at earlier stages, and a noteworthy increase in tumor mutation burden [55]. Furthermore, in the GARNET trial, a limited number of patients with POLE mutations were observed, with the majority of these cases being gastrointestinal cancers. Notably, dostarlimab treatment demonstrated a promising response in this specific population. Patients with microsatellite stable CRC carrying POLE or POLD-1 mutations may exhibit an increased likelihood of benefiting from immunotherapy.

3. Non-targeted therapies

3.1 Chemotherapy rechallenge or reintroduction

Chemotherapy rechallange therapy can be defined as the readministration of a treatment that was previously used but discontinued due to reasons such as toxicity, patient choice, and especially disease progression, after receiving at least one different treatment regimen. Reintroduction is defined as using the same treatment regimen again after discontinuation of treatment without previous disease progression. It is frequently preferred by clinicians, especially in patients receiving multiple serial treatments and in cases where accessible treatment options are reduced. Its efficacy in mCRC has been discussed for a long time. Many studies with positive results have been published [42, 56, 57]. Careful selection of patients, especially when choosing the rechallenge approach in the third step, should take into account their disease burden and residual toxicity. There are many studies showing clinical benefit in appropriate patients [58]. There are also small group studies showing increased efficacy of chemotherapy rechallenge after regorafenib [59]. Briefly, rechallange strategy may be an important treatment option in patients eligible for standard chemotherapy when treatment options are limited, taking into account performance status, previous treatment response, and especially residual toxicities.

3.2 Regorafenib

Regorafenib (BAY 73–4506) is an orally available small-molecule multikinase inhibitor. It inhibits angiogenic kinases (VEGFR1–2-3, platelet-derived growth factor receptor α (PDGFRα) and fibroblast growth factor receptor 1 (FGFR-1)) and mutant oncogenic kinases KIT, RET, and BRAF. It shows antitumoral effect through these mechanisms [60]. The effect of regorafenib on mCRC was first demonstrated in the CORRECT study, an international, multicenter, phase 3 trial. Patients with mCRC who had progression during or within 3 months of the last standard treatment were randomized. A total of 74% of patients received 3 or more serial treatments. Median overall survival was 6.4 months (IQR 3.6–11.8) in the regorafenib group and 5.0 months (IQR 2.8–10.4) in the placebo group. The HR for overall survival was 0.77 [95% CI 0.64–0.94; $p = 0.0052$]. Median PFS was 1.9 months in the regorafenib group (IQR 1.6–3.9) and 1.7 months in the placebo group (1.4–1.9). The HR for PFS was 0.49 [95% CI 0–42–0-58; $p < 0.0001$] for regorafenib vs. placebo [61]. After regorafenib entered daily routine use, studies showing real-life data were conducted. In one of the most important of these studies, the CONCUR study, the real-life data and side effect profile of regorafenib in the Asian population were presented in more details. In this study, median overall survival was 8.8 months [95% CI 7.3–9.8] in the regorafenib group and 6.3 months [95% CI 4.8–7.6] in the placebo group. Overall survival was significantly better with regorafenib than with placebo (HR 0.55, [95% CI 0.40–0-77p = 0–00016]). The most common side effects were hand-foot skin reaction (73%), hyperbilirubinemia (36%), alanine aminotransferase concentration and aspartate aminotransferase concentration increased (24%), and hypertension (23%) as well [62].

3.2.1 Trifluridin ve tipirasil hidroklorürden (TAS-102)

Trifluridine (FTD) and tipiracil hydrochloride (TPI), also known as TAS-102, is an oral antimetabolic agent. FTD is a thymidine-based nucleoside analog, which is incorporated into DNA in the form of triphosphate, causing single-strand and double-strand breaks. TPI is a potent thymidine phosphorylase inhibitor. It prevents the rapid degradation of FTD, and thus ensures a sustained high concentration of FTD after oral administration [63]. In 2015, the RECOURSE study, the results of which were published in 2015, demonstrated its efficacy in mCRC. The RECOURSE study, a randomized phase 3 trial, included 800 patients with mCRC who had received at least two series of standard chemotherapy and had progressed in the last 3 months. The FTD/TPI arm was compared with the placebo arm. Median OS was 7.1 months [95% CI, 6.5–7.8] in the FTD/TPI arm and 5.3 months [95% CI, 4.6–6.0] in the placebo arm. The HR for mortality for FTD/TPI compared with placebo was 0.68 [95% CI, 0.58–0.81; P < 0.001]. Median PFS was 2.0 months [95% CI, 1.9–2.1] in the FTD/TPI arm and 1.7 months [95% CI, 1.7–1.8] in the placebo arm. The HR for progression (FTD/TPI vs. placebo) was 0.48 [95% CI, 0.41–0.57; P < 0.001]. A total of 38% patients had neutropenia, 21% had leukopenia, and 4% had febrile neutropenia [64]. After the RECOURSE study, the results of the C-TASK FORCE study, a phase 1–2 study, were published in 2017. This study compared the use of FTD/TPI alone versus in combination with bevacizumab. After a median follow-up of 10 months, the median PFS was 2.6 months for trifluridine-tipiracil alone and 4.6 months in combination with bevacizumab [HR, 0.45; 95% CI, 0.29–0.72; P = .0015]. These results showed that the use of FTD/TPI with bevacizumab was more effective than its use alone [65]. SUNLİGHT trial, phase 3, international, prospective, randomized, active-controlled, and trial involving patients with refractory metastatic colorectal cancer showed that treatment with FTD–TPI plus bevacizumab resulted in significantly longer overall survival and progression-free survival and better disease control than treatment with FTD–TPI alone. Although a minority of patients did not receive the trial treatment as third-line therapy, this trial was predominantly a third-line trial (>90% of patients had received two previous lines of therapy). The duration of overall survival in the FTD–TPI group was consistent with previous observations, a finding that suggests the benefits observed with FTD–TPI plus bevacizumab will be applicable to all suitable patients with refractory disease [66]. In conclusion, FTD/TPI, both alone and in combination with bevacizumab, improves OS and PFS in patients with mCRC who have received multiple series of treatment. Since combined use with bevacizumab is more effective than monotherapy, combined use may be preferred.

3.2.2 Fruquintinib (HMPL-013)

Fruquintinib (HMPL-013) is a novel oral small molecule that selectively inhibits vascular endothelial growth factor receptors 1, 2, and 3 and has potent inhibitory effects on multiple human tumor xenografts [67]. Its efficacy in patients with mCRC who had received at least 2 prior lines of therapy was examined in the FRESCO study, a phase 3 trial. Median overall survival was significantly prolonged with fruquintinib compared with placebo (9.3 months [95% CI, 8.2–10.5] vs. 6.6 months [95% CI, 5.9–8.1]); the hazard ratio (HR) for mortality was 0.65 (95% CI, 0.51–0.83; P < .001). Median progression-free survival was also significantly increased with fruquintinib (3.7 months [95% CI, 3.7–4.6] vs. 1.8 months [95% CI, 1.8–1.8]); HR for progression or mortality was 0.26 (95% CI, 0.21 to 0.34; P < .001) [68]. The FRESCO-2 study was then conducted, again comparing the fruquintinib arm with the placebo arm. Patients with mCRC included in the study had previously received a median of four lines (IQR 3–6) of systemic therapy and 502 of 691 patients (73%) received more than three lines. Median overall survival was 7.4 months (95% CI 6.7–8.2) in the fruquintinib group vs. 4.8 months in the placebo group ([95% CI 4.0–5.8], HR 0.66, [95% CI 0.55–0.80; p < 0.0001)], PFS was 3.7 months in the fruquintinib arm and 1.8 months in the placebo arm (HR 0.32; [95% CI: 0.27–0.39]; p < 0.001). Side effects seen in the fruquintinib arms in the FRESCO and FRESCO two studies were similar. Grade 3 and above toxicity was seen in more than 60% in both studies. Arterial hypertension was the most common, while hand-foot skin reaction, asthenia, and proteinuria may be observed [69]. Fruquintinib was approved for use in previously treated mCRC by the United States Food and Drug Administration (FDA) in November 2023. Fruquintinib dose is 5 mg orally once daily, for the first 21 days of each 28-day cycle until disease progression or unacceptable toxicity. Despite the elevated occurrence of Grade 3 and above toxicity, signifying the need for caution regarding potential side effects during fruquintinib use, it has emerged as a significant therapeutic option for patients who have undergone multiple sequential treatments.

4. Brief recommendations from guidelines

4.1 ESMO recommendations

The European Society for Medical Oncology (ESMO) metastatic colorectal cancer guideline was last updated in October 2022. In mCRC patients, the approach recommendations in the first, second, and third treatment steps were clearly separated. Since the previous sections mentioned the recommendations for first- and second-line treatments, here, we will only talk about the recommended treatment approaches in the third line and beyond. If progression did not develop during first-line indication therapy, it was suggested that the same treatment could be given as reintroduction after the second series. Single-agent anti-EGFR (panitumumab or cetuximab) was recommended if RAS/BRAF wild patients were not previously treated with anti-EGFR. In RAS/BRAF wild irinotecan-refractory patients, the combination of irinotecan plus cetuximab was recommended more strongly than single-agent cetuximab. The use of another anti-EGFR was not recommended in patients who had previously progressed under anti-EGFR. Dual HER2 blockade was recommended in RAS/BRAF wild-HER2 positive patients. Based on the HERACLES study, the combination of trastuzumab and lapatinib was among the recommendations. The combination of encorafenib and cetuximab was recommended as the best option in series three in patients with previously treated BRAF V600E-mutated mCRC. In all patients, regardless of RAS/BRAF status, the oral agents reegorafenib or trifluridineetipiracil (TAS-102), which have previously shown superiority over BSC, were recommended. It is noteworthy that immunotherapy options (pembrolizumab, nivolumab, ipilimumab, and nivolumab) were recommended in the first- and second-line setting rather than third-line setting [70].

4.2 NCCN recommendations

First, NCCN divided patients into two groups: pMMR/MSS and dMMR/MSI-H. In the dMMR/MSI-H patient group, checkpoint inhibitor immunotherapy (pembrolizumab, nivolumab, nivolumab plus ipilimumab, or dostarlimab-gxly) was recommended as the first line of treatment. In patients who progressed under immunotherapy, systemic therapies were recommended in the next-line treatments. Cetuximab or panitumumab ±irinotecan treatment was recommended in the third step in patients with KRAS/NRAS/BRAF wild type located only in the left arm who had not received anti-EGFR therapy before. Cetuximab or panitumumab ±irinotecan treatment in the third line was suggested to be used in patients who received irinotecan-based treatment in the first series plus oxaliplatin-based treatment + anti-EGFR in the second series. However, emphasizing the number of patients and patient distribution of the studies on rechallenge, rechallenge was not recommended for treatment regimens under which progression had previously occurred. However, it was suggested that treatments that were discontinued due to conditions, such as adjuvant therapy, cumulative toxicity, treatment break, and patient preference, could be reintroduced in advanced steps. In the pMMR/MSS patient group, fruquintinib, regorafenib, trifluridine + tipiracil ± bevacizumab (primarily in combination with bevacizumab) treatments were recommended regardless of any mutation status in patients who received standard treatment in previous series [71].

4.3 ASCO recommendations

The ASCO guideline was last updated in October 2022. For this, the most recent treatments such as fruquintinib, sotorasib, and adagrasib were not included. Pembrolizumab treatment was recommended in MSH patients. Standard chemotherapy and anti-VEGFs were recommended in RAS mutant patients.

Standard chemotherapy and anti-EGFR antibodies were recommended in RAS/BRAF wild patients with left colon localization. Encorafenib plus cetuximab was recommended in BRAF V600E mutant patients with progression who had received at least one prior series of treatment [72].

5. Summary

Discoveries in tumor biology and advances in molecular diagnostic methods help to determine the most appropriate approach to treatment by analyzing the genetic structure of tumors of patients with mCRC in detail. This increases the importance of personalized treatment strategies in the treatment of advanced stages of mCRC. The dMMR/MSI-H status of the tumor, HER2 amplification or overexpression, KRAS 12C mutation, NTRK mutation, RET mutation, BRAF/MET status, TMB or POLE mutation status are prominent in evaluating treatment options.

Pembrolizumab, dostalizumab, nivolumab, and nivolumab plus ipilimumab treatments may be preferred in patients with dMMR/MSI-H if immunotherapy option was not used in previous lines. In particular, nivolumab plus ipilimumab treatment is ahead of the other treatments with an ORR of 65%, but dostalimab also draws attention with an ORR of 43.5%.

Trastuzumab and pertuzumab, trastuzumab and tucatinib, trastuzumab deruxtecan (T-DXd), trastuzumab and lapatinib may be preferred in patients with HER2 amplification or overexpression. Among these treatment options, trastuzumab+tucatinib treatment seems to be more prominent than other treatment options with higher ORR, PFS, and OS values.

Although adagrasib and sotorasib monotherapies have shown their efficacy in patients with KRAS 12C mutation, better survival results have been obtained in combination with anti-EGFR. Therefore, the preference for combined use in KRAS 12C mutant patients will be a more accurate approach than monotherapies.

Larotrectinib and entrectinib in solid tumors with NTRK fusion, and selpercatinib in patients with RET fusion have been approved for tumor-agnostic use, but the number of patients with mCRC in these studies is quite small. and it seems clear that new studies are needed to support the data. Encorafenib and cetuximab or panitumumab and/or binimetinib have demonstrated safety in terms of efficacy and side effect profile in patients with BRAF V600E mutated mCRC.

Regorafenib, trifluridine and tipiracil hydrochloride (TAS-102), fruquintinib have been replaced by regorafenib, Trifluridine and tipiracil hydrochloride (TAS-102) in patients who are not suitable for targeted therapies or who do not respond to these therapies. While regorafenib and fruquintinib are used as monotherapy, TAS-102 can be used as monotherapy or in combination with bevacizumab. Bevacizumab combination gives better results compared to monotherapy.

In cases where accessible treatment options are reduced, the use of conventional chemotherapies as rechallenge or reintroduction is frequently preferred by clinicians. They can also be used in patients who cannot be controlled with targetable agents. In addition, conventional chemotherapies are indispensable for many clinicians when financial toxicities are considered.

Despite all these developments, treatment responses and survival rates show that new developments are still needed in this field.

Conflict of interest

The authors declare no conflict of interest.

Author details

Ali Kaan Güren and Osman Köstek*
Division of Medical Oncology, Department of Medical Oncology, Marmara University School of Medicine, Istanbul, Turkey

*Address all correspondence to: osmankostek@hotmail.com

References

[1] Siegel RL, Giaquinto AN, Jemal A. Cancer statistics, 2024. CA: a Cancer Journal for Clinicians. 2024;**74**(1):12-49

[2] Society TAC. Survival rates for colorectal cancer. In: Cancer Facts & Figures 2024. American Cancer Society; 2024. Available from: https://www.cancer.org/cancer/types/colon-rectal-cancer/detection-diagnosis-staging/survival-rates.html

[3] Nader Hanna CW, Zheng Z, Onukwugha E, Seal BS, Mullins CD. Survival benefit associated with the number of chemotherapy/biologic treatment lines in 5,129 metastatic colon cancer patients. Journal of Clinical Oncology. 2014;**32**:559. DOI: 10.1200/jco.2014.32.3_suppl.559

[4] Tampellini M, Di Maio M, Baratelli C, Anania L, Brizzi MP, Sonetto C, et al. Treatment of patients with metastatic colorectal cancer in a real-world scenario: Probability of receiving second and further lines of therapy and description of clinical benefit. Clinical Colorectal Cancer. 2017;**16**(4):372-376

[5] Buchler T. Microsatellite instability and metastatic colorectal cancer - a clinical perspective. Frontiers in Oncology. 2022;**12**:888181

[6] Le DT, Kim TW, Van Cutsem E, Geva R, Jäger D, Hara H, et al. Phase II open-label study of pembrolizumab in treatment-refractory, microsatellite instability-high/mismatch repair-deficient metastatic colorectal cancer: KEYNOTE-164. Journal of Clinical Oncology. 2020;**38**(1):11-19

[7] Overman MJ, McDermott R, Leach JL, Lonardi S, Lenz HJ, Morse MA, et al. Nivolumab in patients with metastatic DNA mismatch repair-deficient or microsatellite instability-high colorectal cancer (CheckMate 142): An open-label, multicentre, phase 2 study. The Lancet Oncology. 2017;**18**(9):1182-1191

[8] André T, Lonardi S, Wong KYM, Lenz HJ, Gelsomino F, Aglietta M, et al. Nivolumab plus low-dose ipilimumab in previously treated patients with microsatellite instability-high/mismatch repair-deficient metastatic colorectal cancer: 4-year follow-up from CheckMate 142. Annals of Oncology. 2022;**33**(10):1052-1060

[9] Markham A. Dostarlimab: First approval. Drugs. 2021;**81**(10):1213-1219

[10] Oaknin A, Pothuri B, Gilbert L, Sabatier R, Brown J, Ghamande S, et al. Safety, Efficacy, and Biomarker Analyses of Dostarlimab in Patients with Endometrial Cancer: Interim Results of the Phase I GARNET Study. Clinical Cancer Research. 14 Nov 2023;**29**(22):4564-4574. DOI: 10.1158/1078-0432.CCR-22-3915. PMID: 37363992; PMCID: PMC10643997

[11] André T, Berton D, Curigliano G, Sabatier R, Tinker AV, Oaknin A, et al. Antitumor activity and safety of dostarlimab monotherapy in patients with mismatch repair deficient solid tumors: A nonrandomized controlled trial. JAMA Network Open. 2023;**6**(11):e2341165

[12] Ross JS, Fakih M, Ali SM, Elvin JA, Schrock AB, Suh J, et al. Targeting HER2 in colorectal cancer: The landscape of amplification and short variant mutations in ERBB2 and ERBB3. Cancer. 2018;**124**(7):1358-1373

[13] Meric-Bernstam F, Hurwitz H, Raghav KPS, McWilliams RR, Fakih M, Vander Walde A, et al. Pertuzumab

plus trastuzumab for HER2-amplified metastatic colorectal cancer (MyPathway): An updated report from a multicentre, open-label, phase 2a, multiple basket study. The Lancet Oncology. 2019;**20**(4):518-530

[14] Zheng-Lin B, Bekaii-Saab TS. Treatment options for HER2-expressing colorectal cancer: Updates and recent approvals. Therapeutic Advances in Medical Oncology. 2024;**16**:17588359231225037

[15] Chitkara A, Bakhtiar M, Sahin IH, Hsu D, Zhang J, Anamika F, et al. A meta-analysis to assess the efficacy of HER2-targeted treatment regimens in HER2-positive metastatic colorectal cancer (mCRC). Current Oncology. 2023;**30**(9):8266-8277

[16] Gupta R, Meric-Bernstam F, Rothe M, Garrett-Mayer E, Mangat PK, D'Andre S, et al. Pertuzumab plus Trastuzumab in patients with colorectal cancer with ERBB2 amplification or ERBB2/3 mutations: Results from the TAPUR study. JCO Precision Oncology. 2022;**6**:e2200306

[17] Yoshikawa A, Nakamura Y. Treatment strategies for HER2-positive metastatic colorectal cancer. Gan to Kagaku Ryoho. 2023;**50**(7):763-767

[18] Kulukian A, Lee P, Taylor J, Rosler R, de Vries P, Watson D, et al. Preclinical activity of HER2-selective tyrosine kinase inhibitor tucatinib as a single agent or in combination with trastuzumab or docetaxel in solid tumor models. Molecular Cancer Therapeutics. 2020;**19**(4):976-987

[19] Strickler JH, Cercek A, Siena S, André T, Ng K, Van Cutsem E, et al. Tucatinib plus trastuzumab for chemotherapy-refractory, HER2-positive, RAS wild-type unresectable or metastatic colorectal cancer (MOUNTAINEER): A multicentre, open-label, phase 2 study. The Lancet Oncology. 2023;**24**(5):496-508

[20] Iwata TN, Ishii C, Ishida S, Ogitani Y, Wada T, Agatsuma T. A HER2-targeting antibody-drug conjugate, trastuzumab deruxtecan (DS-8201a), enhances antitumor immunity in a mouse model. Molecular Cancer Therapeutics. 2018;**17**(7):1494-1503

[21] Yoshino T, Di Bartolomeo M, Raghav K, Masuishi T, Loupakis F, Kawakami H, et al. Final results of DESTINY-CRC01 investigating trastuzumab deruxtecan in patients with HER2-expressing metastatic colorectal cancer. Nature Communications. 2023;**14**(1):3332

[22] Nelson MH, Dolder CR. Lapatinib: A novel dual tyrosine kinase inhibitor with activity in solid tumors. The Annals of Pharmacotherapy. 2006;**40**(2):261-269

[23] Sartore-Bianchi A, Trusolino L, Martino C, Bencardino K, Lonardi S, Bergamo F, et al. Dual-targeted therapy with trastuzumab and lapatinib in treatment-refractory, KRAS codon 12/13 wild-type, HER2-positive metastatic colorectal cancer (HERACLES): A proof-of-concept, multicentre, open-label, phase 2 trial. The Lancet Oncology. 2016;**17**(6):738-746

[24] Awad MM, Liu S, Rybkin II, Arbour KC, Dilly J, Zhu VW, et al. Acquired resistance to KRAS(G12C) inhibition in cancer. The New England Journal of Medicine. 2021;**384**(25):2382-2393

[25] Fakih MG, Kopetz S, Kuboki Y, Kim TW, Munster PN, Krauss JC, et al. Sotorasib for previously treated colorectal cancers with KRAS(G12C) mutation (CodeBreaK100): A prespecified analysis

of a single-arm, phase 2 trial. The Lancet Oncology. 2022;**23**(1):115-124

[26] Fakih MG, Salvatore L, Esaki T, Modest DP, Lopez-Bravo DP, Taieb J, et al. Sotorasib plus panitumumab in refractory colorectal cancer with mutated KRAS G12C. The New England Journal of Medicine. 2023;**389**(23):2125-2139

[27] Bekaii-Saab TS, Yaeger R, Spira AI, Pelster MS, Sabari JK, Hafez N, et al. Adagrasib in advanced solid tumors harboring a KRAS(G12C) mutation. Journal of Clinical Oncology. 2023;**41**(25):4097-4106

[28] Yaeger R, Weiss J, Pelster MS, Spira AI, Barve M, Ou SI, et al. Adagrasib with or without cetuximab in colorectal cancer with mutated KRAS G12C. The New England Journal of Medicine. 2023;**388**(1):44-54

[29] Gatalica Z, Xiu J, Swensen J, Vranic S. Molecular characterization of cancers with NTRK gene fusions. Modern Pathology. 2019;**32**(1):147-153

[30] Wang H, Li ZW, Ou Q, Wu X, Nagasaka M, Shao Y, et al. NTRK fusion positive colorectal cancer is a unique subset of CRC with high TMB and microsatellite instability. Cancer Medicine. 2022;**11**(13):2541-2549

[31] Dunn DB. Larotrectinib and entrectinib: TRK inhibitors for the treatment of pediatric and adult patients with NTRK gene fusion. Journal of the Advanced Practitioner in Oncology. 2020;**11**(4):418-423

[32] Carlson JJ, Italiano A, Brose MS, Federman N, Lassen U, Kummar S, et al. Comparative effectiveness of larotrectinib and entrectinib for TRK fusion cancer. The American Journal of Managed Care. 2022;**28**(2 Suppl):S26-s32

[33] Drilon A, Laetsch TW, Kummar S, DuBois SG, Lassen UN, Demetri GD, et al. Efficacy of larotrectinib in TRK fusion-positive cancers in adults and children. The New England Journal of Medicine. 2018;**378**(8):731-739

[34] Santos C, Sanz-Pamplona R, Salazar R. RET-fusions: a novel paradigm in colorectal cancer. Annals of Oncology. 2018;**29**(6):1340-1343

[35] Jhiang SM. The RET proto-oncogene in human cancers. Oncogene. 2000;**19**(49):5590-5597

[36] Le Rolle AF, Klempner SJ, Garrett CR, Seery T, Sanford EM, Balasubramanian S, et al. Identification and characterization of RET fusions in advanced colorectal cancer. Oncotarget. 2015;**6**(30):28929-28937

[37] Pietrantonio F, Di Nicolantonio F, Schrock AB, Lee J, Tejpar S, Sartore-Bianchi A, et al. ALK, ROS1, and NTRK Rearrangements in Metastatic Colorectal Cancer. Journal of the National Cancer Institute. 1 Dec 2017;**109**(12). DOI: 10.1093/jnci/djx089. PMID: 29370427

[38] Duke ES, Bradford D, Marcovitz M, Amatya AK, Mishra-Kalyani PS, Nguyen E, et al. FDA approval summary: Selpercatinib for the treatment of advanced RET fusion-positive solid tumors. Clinical Cancer Research. 2023;**29**(18):3573-3578

[39] Subbiah V, Wolf J, Konda B, Kang H, Spira A, Weiss J, et al. Tumour-agnostic efficacy and safety of selpercatinib in patients with RET fusion-positive solid tumours other than lung or thyroid tumours (LIBRETTO-001): A phase 1/2, open-label, basket trial. The Lancet Oncology. 2022;**23**(10):1261-1273

[40] Sidaway P. From AACR 2022. Nature Reviews. Clinical Oncology. 2022;**19**(6):359

[41] Schulz MS, Wolf S, Struck V, Thomas N, Husman G, Zeuzem S, et al. Anti-EGFR reintroduction and rechallenge in metastatic colorectal cancer (mCRC): A real-world analysis. Cancers (Basel). 2022;**14**(7):1641

[42] Cremolini C, Rossini D, Dell'Aquila E, Lonardi S, Conca E, Del Re M, et al. Rechallenge for patients with RAS and BRAF wild-type metastatic colorectal cancer with acquired resistance to first-line cetuximab and irinotecan: A phase 2 single-arm clinical trial. JAMA Oncology. 2019;**5**(3):343-350

[43] Martinelli E, Martini G, Famiglietti V, Troiani T, Napolitano S, Pietrantonio F, et al. Cetuximab rechallenge plus avelumab in pretreated patients with RAS wild-type metastatic colorectal cancer: The phase 2 single-arm clinical CAVE trial. JAMA Oncology. 2021;**7**(10):1529-1535

[44] Sartore-Bianchi A, Pietrantonio F, Lonardi S, Mussolin B, Rua F, Crisafulli G, et al. Circulating tumor DNA to guide rechallenge with panitumumab in metastatic colorectal cancer: The phase 2 CHRONOS trial. Nature Medicine. 2022;**28**(8):1612-1618

[45] Rossini D, Germani MM, Lonardi S, Pietrantonio F, Dell'Aquila E, Borelli B, et al. Treatments after second progression in metastatic colorectal cancer: A pooled analysis of the TRIBE and TRIBE2 studies. European Journal of Cancer. 2022;**170**:64-72

[46] Cohen R, Liu H, Fiskum J, Adams R, Chibaudel B, Maughan TS, et al. BRAF V600E mutation in first-line metastatic colorectal cancer: An analysis of individual patient data from the ARCAD database. Journal of the National Cancer Institute. 2021;**113**(10):1386-1395

[47] Kim G, McKee AE, Ning YM, Hazarika M, Theoret M, Johnson JR, et al. FDA approval summary: Vemurafenib for treatment of unresectable or metastatic melanoma with the BRAFV600E mutation. Clinical Cancer Research. 2014;**20**(19):4994-5000

[48] Kopetz S, Guthrie KA, Morris VK, Lenz HJ, Magliocco AM, Maru D, et al. Randomized trial of irinotecan and cetuximab with or without vemurafenib in BRAF-mutant metastatic colorectal cancer (SWOG S1406). Journal of Clinical Oncology. 2021;**39**(4):285-294

[49] Koelblinger P, Thuerigen O, Dummer R. Development of encorafenib for BRAF-mutated advanced melanoma. Current Opinion in Oncology. 2018;**30**(2):125-133

[50] Wu PK, Park JI. MEK1/2 inhibitors: Molecular activity and resistance mechanisms. Seminars in Oncology. 2015;**42**(6):849-862

[51] Kopetz S, Grothey A, Yaeger R, Van Cutsem E, Desai J, Yoshino T, et al. Encorafenib, binimetinib, and cetuximab in BRAF V600E-mutated colorectal cancer. The New England Journal of Medicine. 2019;**381**(17):1632-1643

[52] Fancello L, Gandini S, Pelicci PG, Mazzarella L. Tumor mutational burden quantification from targeted gene panels: Major advancements and challenges. Journal for Immunotherapy of Cancer. 2019;7(1):183

[53] Marabelle A, Fakih M, Lopez J, Shah M, Shapira-Frommer R, Nakagawa K, et al. Association of tumour mutational burden with outcomes in patients with advanced solid tumours treated with pembrolizumab: Prospective biomarker analysis of the multicohort, open-label, phase 2 KEYNOTE-158 study. The Lancet Oncology. 2020;**21**(10):1353-1365

[54] Meiri E, Garrett-Mayer E, Halabi S, Mangat P, Shrestha S, Ahn E, et al. Pembrolizumab (P) in patients (pts) with colorectal cancer (CRC) with high tumor mutational burden (HTMB): Results from the targeted agent and profiling utilization registry (TAPUR) study. Journal of Clinical Oncology. 2020;**38**:133

[55] Hu H, Cai W, Wu D, Hu W, Dong Wang L, Mao J, et al. Ultra-mutated colorectal cancer patients with POLE driver mutations exhibit distinct clinical patterns. Cancer Medicine. 2021;**10**(1):135-142

[56] Costa T, Nuñez J, Felismino T, Boente L, Mello C. REOX: Evaluation of the efficacy of retreatment with an oxaliplatin-containing regimen in metastatic colorectal cancer: A retrospective single-center study. Clinical Colorectal Cancer. 2017;**16**(4):316-323

[57] Liu X, George GC, Tsimberidou AM, Naing A, Wheler JJ, Kopetz S, et al. Retreatment with anti-EGFR based therapies in metastatic colorectal cancer: Impact of intervening time interval and prior anti-EGFR response. BMC Cancer. 2015;**15**:713

[58] Köstek O, Hacıoğlu MB, Sakin A, Demir T, Sarı M, Ozkul O, et al. Regorafenib or rechallenge chemotherapy: Which is more effective in the third-line treatment of metastatic colorectal cancer? Cancer Chemotherapy and Pharmacology. 2019;**83**(1):115-122

[59] Bertocchi P, Aroldi F, Prochilo T, Meriggi F, Beretta GD, Zaniboni A. Chemotherapy rechallenge after regorafenib treatment in metastatic colorectal cancer: Still hope after the last hope? Journal of Chemotherapy. 2017;**29**(2):102-105

[60] Wilhelm SM, Dumas J, Adnane L, Lynch M, Carter CA, Schütz G, et al. Regorafenib (BAY 73-4506): A new oral multikinase inhibitor of angiogenic, stromal and oncogenic receptor tyrosine kinases with potent preclinical antitumor activity. International Journal of Cancer. 2011;**129**(1):245-255

[61] Grothey A, Van Cutsem E, Sobrero A, Siena S, Falcone A, Ychou M, et al. Regorafenib monotherapy for previously treated metastatic colorectal cancer (CORRECT): An international, multicentre, randomised, placebo-controlled, phase 3 trial. Lancet. 2013;**381**(9863):303-312

[62] Li J, Qin S, Xu R, Yau TC, Ma B, Pan H, et al. Regorafenib plus best supportive care versus placebo plus best supportive care in Asian patients with previously treated metastatic colorectal cancer (CONCUR): A randomised, double-blind, placebo-controlled, phase 3 trial. The Lancet Oncology. 2015;**16**(6):619-629

[63] Bendell JC, Rosen LS, Mayer RJ, Goldman JW, Infante JR, Benedetti F, et al. Phase 1 study of oral TAS-102 in patients with refractory metastatic colorectal cancer. Cancer Chemotherapy and Pharmacology. 2015;**76**(5):925-932

[64] Mayer RJ, Van Cutsem E, Falcone A, Yoshino T, Garcia-Carbonero R, Mizunuma N, et al. Randomized trial of TAS-102 for refractory metastatic colorectal cancer. The New England Journal of Medicine. 2015;**372**(20):1909-1919

[65] Kuboki Y, Nishina T, Shinozaki E, Yamazaki K, Shitara K, Okamoto W, et al. TAS-102 plus bevacizumab for patients with metastatic colorectal cancer refractory to standard therapies (C-TASK FORCE): An investigator-initiated, open-label, single-arm, multicentre, phase 1/2 study. The Lancet Oncology. 2017;**18**(9):1172-1181

[66] Prager GW, Taieb J, Fakih M, Ciardiello F, Van Cutsem E, Elez E, et al. Trifluridine-tipiracil and bevacizumab in refractory metastatic colorectal cancer. The New England Journal of Medicine. 2023;**388**(18):1657-1667

[67] Cao J, Zhang J, Peng W, Chen Z, Fan S, Su W, et al. A phase I study of safety and pharmacokinetics of fruquintinib, a novel selective inhibitor of vascular endothelial growth factor receptor-1, -2, and -3 tyrosine kinases in Chinese patients with advanced solid tumors. Cancer Chemotherapy and Pharmacology. 2016;**78**(2):259-269

[68] Li J, Qin S, Xu RH, Shen L, Xu J, Bai Y, et al. Effect of fruquintinib vs placebo on overall survival in patients with previously treated metastatic colorectal cancer: The FRESCO randomized clinical trial. Journal of the American Medical Association. 2018;**319**(24):2486-2496

[69] Dasari A, Lonardi S, Garcia-Carbonero R, Elez E, Yoshino T, Sobrero A, et al. Fruquintinib versus placebo in patients with refractory metastatic colorectal cancer (FRESCO-2): An international, multicentre, randomised, double-blind, phase 3 study. Lancet. 2023;**402**(10395):41-53

[70] Cervantes A, Adam R, Roselló S, Arnold D, Normanno N, Taïeb J, et al. Metastatic colorectal cancer: ESMO clinical practice guideline for diagnosis, treatment and follow-up. Annals of Oncology. 2023;**34**(1):10-32

[71] NCCN. NCCN Clinical Practice Guidelines in Oncology-Colon Cancer Version 4.2023. NCCN; 2023. Available from: http://www.nccn.org/

[72] Morris VK, Kennedy EB, Baxter NN, Benson AB 3rd, Cercek A, Cho M, et al. Treatment of metastatic colorectal cancer: ASCO guideline. Journal of Clinical Oncology. 2023;**41**(3):678-700

Chapter 6

Complications Following Colorectal Cancer Surgery

Veysel Cem Ozcan

Abstract

Postoperative complications following colorectal cancer surgery occur in approximately 50% of patients, resulting in increased healthcare expenses and a decline in quality of life. Complication classification systems are commonly used to assess and categorize these adverse events across various healthcare institutions. The widely used Clavien-Dindo system is effective in classifying complications based on their clinical severity, yet it does not provide insights into the underlying factors contributing to their occurrence. Another classification system, the American College of Surgeons National Surgical Quality Improvement Program (NSQIP) surgical risk calculator, was developed to accurately predict complications and length of stay. Most current studies primarily focus on the prevention of complications, employing preoperative, intraoperative, and postoperative interventions. Factors such as surgical technique selection, fluid therapy, transfusion preferences, and mechanical bowel cleaning can all play a significant role in reducing the occurrence of complications. Furthermore, patient-associated factors such as age, gender, tumor location, and body mass index (BMI) also influence the likelihood of experiencing complications. Postoperative complications not only negatively impact short-term quality of life and healthcare costs but also have long-term implications on oncological outcomes. These complications can result in delays or discontinuation of chemotherapy, even in patients who have clear indications for systemic therapy.

Keywords: colorectal cancer, surgery, complications, survival, factors affecting complications

1. Introduction

Postoperative complications in patients undergoing colorectal cancer surgery occur in approximately 50% of cases and have been found to be associated with increased rates of morbidity and mortality, elevated healthcare costs, and a decline in overall quality of life.

A study conducted in the United Kingdom examining complications following colorectal surgery revealed that the in-hospital mortality rate ranged from 1 to 6.5%, while mortality within 30 days ranged from 0.7 to 11.3%. Additionally, the study reported a morbidity rate between 26.4 and 54.5%. Similarly, a separate study conducted in the United States, with a comparable objective, observed a mortality rate of 3.9% after colorectal surgery, a general morbidity rate of 24.3%, and a severe morbidity rate of 11.4%.

2. Classification and prediction of complications

Most existing research focuses on the prevention of complications, and several classification systems have been developed for this purpose. Among these systems, the Clavien-Dindo classification system stands out as the most useful. This system allows for easy comparison of complications across different time periods within the same institution, as well as between different institutions. Furthermore, it enables the comparison of surgical and conservative treatments, standardized documentation of operations, and associated complications and facilitates meta-analysis. However, it is important to note that the Clavien-Dindo classification system does not assess pre-existing conditions and comorbidities, despite their significant role in the occurrence of complications. In the Clavien-Dindo classification, only five grades of postoperative complications are defined (**Table 1**). Another classification system that offers a different approach is the American College of Surgeons National Surgical Quality Improvement Program (NSQIP) surgical risk calculator. This model is built using data from over 4.3 million operations in the ACS NSQIP database. The current Universal Risk Calculator can be used for any procedure, in most surgical subspecialties, while previously developed NSQIP-based risk calculators can only be used for individual procedures (e.g., colectomy, pancreatectomy, etc.). The primary goal of this system is to accurately predict the risk of complications and length of stay for patients. The NSQIP takes into consideration the impact of a patient's comorbidities on the risk

Grade I	Any deviation from the normal postoperative course without the need for pharmacological treatment or surgical, endoscopic, and radiological interventions. Allowed therapeutic regimens are drugs as antiemetics, antipyretics, analgetics, diuretics, electrolytes, and physiotherapy. This grade also includes wound infections opened at the bedside.
Grade II	Requiring pharmacological treatment with drugs other than such allowed for grade I complications. Blood transfusions and total parenteral nutrition are also included.
Grade III	Requiring surgical, endoscopic, or radiological intervention
a	Intervention not under general anesthesia
b	Intervention under general anesthesia
Grade IV	Life-threatening complication (including CNS complications)* requiring IC/ICU management
a	Single organ dysfunction (including dialysis)
b	Multiorgan dysfunction
Grade V	Death of a patient
d	If the patient suffers from a complication at the time of discharge, the suffix "d" (for"disability") is added to the respective grade of complication. This label indicates the need for a follow-up to fully evaluate the complication.

**Brain hemorrhage, ischemic stroke, sub-arachnoidal bleeding, but excluding transient ischemic attacks. CNS, central nervous system; IC, intermediate care; ICU, intensive care unit.*

Table 1.
Classification of surgical complications.

of postoperative complications. The calculator is online and accessible available at https://riskcalculator.facs.org/RiskCalculator/index.jsp.

2.1 Operative procedures in colorectal cancer and their effect on complications

The surgical techniques used in the management of colorectal malignancies can be categorized into three main types: open surgery, laparoscopic surgery, and robotic surgery. Recently, there has been a significant advancement in endoscopic interventions, leading to the inclusion of therapeutic endoscopic approaches as a distinct group in the treatment of colorectal malignancies.

Several publications have explored the impact of different surgical techniques on the occurrence of complications. Comparing open surgery to laparoscopic surgery, the latter has been found to offer several advantages, including smaller incision length, reduced blood loss, and decreased post-operative pain. However, it should be noted that, for larger tumors, laparoscopic surgery may be less effective due to limitations in traction, resulting in inadequate exploration [1].

Laparoscopic surgery is associated with reduced blood loss when compared to open surgery. This difference can be attributed to the implementation of a high-resolution camera system during laparoscopic procedures, which allows for enhanced visualization and the ability to thoroughly examine multiple anatomical areas.

The findings of the MRC CLASICC study indicated that patients who underwent laparoscopic surgery had a shorter hospital stay compared to those who had the open surgical approach. Furthermore, the study found no significant variation in the occurrence of complications among the two groups at both 30 days and 3 months post-surgery.

Various comparative effectiveness studies investigating the laparoscopic approach versus the open approach in colon surgery have consistently demonstrated that minimally invasive techniques yield better short-term outcomes.

3. Intraoperative complications

The complications observed during colorectal surgery can be identified as follows: bleeding, injury to the small intestine and colon, vascular injuries, ureter and bladder injury, seminal vesicle injury, vaginal injury, splenic injury, presacral bleeding, and pelvic nerve injury.

3.1 Presacral hemorrhage

Preservation of the presacral fascia during rectal mobilization is crucial in preventing such complications. In the event of a ruptured presacral vein, severe bleeding occurs; however, it can effectively be controlled through suturing or cauterization.

3.2 Splenic injury

Iatrogenic splenic laceration is a frequent occurrence in colorectal surgery, often seen during left colon mobilization. Typically, the injury is limited, manifesting as a capsular tear on the anterior and inner surface of the spleen's lower pole, resulting from traction on the splenic ligaments or greater omentum. In instances where the greater omentum is pulled, the injury may extend to the splenic hilum. In the past, splenectomy was commonly performed in all types of splenic injuries; however, recent recommendations suggest prioritizing spleen preservation whenever feasible. To prevent bleeding caused by splenic capsule tears, local hemostatic agents or electrocoagulation can be employed. If uncertainty persists despite these measures, splenectomy remains the most appropriate procedure.

3.3 Ureter, bladder, and urethra injuries

Intraoperative iatrogenic urethral injuries can occur when pelvic anatomy is disrupted due to factors such as pelvic inflammation, previous surgical interventions, radiation therapy, or malignancy. The occurrence rate of iatrogenic ureteral injury in colorectal surgery ranges from 0.3 to 1.5%. However, only a small number of these injuries are actually identified during the surgical procedure itself. The suspicion of an injury can be confirmed through various diagnostic methods including intravenous pyelogram (IVP), retrograde injection of methylene blue, intravenous administration of methylene blue or indigo carmine, or the administration of contrast material through a ureteral catheter.

Timely recognition and repair of an injury significantly enhance the recovery process. Late diagnosis, on the other hand, leads to substantial morbidity and increases the likelihood of nephrectomy by seven times. In the context of colon surgeries, it is noteworthy that injuries to the left ureter are more prevalent compared to the right ureter.

Risk factors that contribute to bladder injury during colorectal surgery encompass a range of factors such as previous surgeries, radiation therapy, malignant infiltration, chronic infections, and inflammatory conditions. To diagnose such injuries radiologically, healthcare professionals typically utilize either a CT cystogram or a fluoroscopic cystogram. In cases where minor extraperitoneal injuries are identified, repair is necessary, and the condition can be effectively treated through a period of 7–14 days with foley catheter decompression.

Among intraoperative urologic injuries, damage to the urethra is considered the least common. This type of injury frequently arises during abdominoperineal resection procedures. Fistula or stricture formation is a typical complication associated with such injuries. To accurately locate the site of injury, medical professionals rely on various diagnostic methods including cystoscopy, retrograde urethrogram, examination under anesthesia, and CT scan with both oral and rectal contrast. The preferred approach for management involves a double primary repair utilizing absorbable sutures at the time of injury. Additionally, utilizing an omental flap or a local tissue flap may help reduce the likelihood of postoperative fistula development.

4. Postoperative complications

Postoperative complications can be classified into two categories based on their occurrence in the early or late postoperative period. Early and late complications are closely interconnected clinical parameters. The early postoperative period is associated with the development of anastomotic leakage, anastomotic bleeding, and stenosis, in addition to postoperative ileus. In the case of inflammatory bowel diseases, there is a higher prevalence of thromboembolism and portal vein thrombosis. In the early postoperative period, hollow organ injuries may present with symptoms. Furthermore, wound complications, surgical site infections, and perineal complications can also arise during this period. On the other hand, in the late postoperative period, one may encounter complications related to stomas. Peristomal infection and skin problems may manifest as early clinical symptoms during this period.

4.1 Ileus

Postoperative ileus refers to the transient loss of intestinal motor function that typically occurs after abdominal surgery. This response is triggered by the stimulation of splanchnic sympathetic nerves as a result of bowel manipulation during the surgical procedure. However, it can also be seen following surgery or trauma to other organs. Gastric atony, which is the loss of muscle tone in the stomach, usually resolves within one to 2 hours. The small intestine recovers its normal motor function within 1–2 days, while the large intestine takes approximately 2–3 days. It may take up to 5 days for the resumption of regular motor function in the intestines following postoperative ileus.

In the context of intra-abdominal infection, it is important to address the underlying cause in order to resolve persistent ileus. Symptoms such as fever, leukocytosis, and abdominal pain may suggest the presence of intra-abdominal infection or anastomotic leakage. To address this condition, certain measures should be implemented. These include the use of a nasogastric tube for decompression, suitable intravenous fluid replacement, administration of antiemetic and prokinetic agents, and correction of any electrolyte imbalances.

4.2 Bladder dysfunction

Bladder dysfunction is a frequently encountered issue that arises when the parasympathetic nerves responsible for innervating the detrusor muscle or the sympathetic nerves responsible for innervating the bladder neck, trigone, and urethra sustain damage during pelvic dissection. This condition can be further exacerbated by postoperative distension, prostatic hypertrophy, and pain. Following rectal dissection, bladder dysfunction has been observed to occur in approximately 20–30% of cases. However, it is important to note that the majority of patients gradually regain their bladder emptying capabilities, although this recovery process may take up to six months.

4.3 Sexual dysfunction

Sexual dysfunction can result from damage to the sympathetic and parasympathetic nerves in the pelvic region. Studies have reported a wide range of prevalence rates, with sexual dysfunction occurring in approximately 15–60% of cases. The parasympathetic erigentes nerves are responsible for the neurological impulse that triggers an erection, while the sympathetic nerves are involved in the neurological impulse for ejaculation. It is worth noting that female patients are generally less likely to experience sexual dysfunction in comparison to their male counterparts.

Here is evidence to suggest that sexual dysfunction following proctectomy may show spontaneous improvement within 6–12 months post-surgery. Additionally, the use of sildenafil has shown promising results in improving erectile dysfunction in approximately 80% of patients. Notably, the use of sildenafil may also contribute to reducing postoperative morbidity [2].

4.4 Fecal incontinence

Following an inferior anterior resection procedure, a small percentage of patients (approximately 5–6%) may experience the development of fecal incontinence, an increased number of bowel movements, and a decrease in the overall quality of life. The causes of anal sphincter dysfunction in these cases are multifactorial. Possible factors include damage to the sphincter caused by anastomotic staples applied through the anus or denervation of the pelvic muscles during rectal mobilization. However, it is important to note that these dysfunctions have the potential to improve within one-year post-surgery.

4.5 Femoral and peroneal neuropathies

Automatic retractors have been identified as a common cause of femoral neuropathies. The reported incidence of femoral neuropathy following colon resection is approximately 0.7%. The femoral nerve, as the largest branch of the lumbar plexus, can potentially be injured during the passage through the psoas muscle. Patients experiencing this condition may present with symptoms such as weakness of the quadriceps femoris, reduced or absent patellar tendon reflexes, and hypoesthesia of the anteromedial thigh. However, the prognosis for femoral neuropathy is generally positive, with over 90% of patients showing recovery through the implementation of physical therapy.

4.6 Thromboembolism

The occurrence rate of thromboembolic events typically ranges from 1 to 7%. Although many deep vein thromboses do not show symptoms, they can occasionally progress to pulmonary embolism, which carries the risk of fatality. Findings from various randomized trials indicate that the preventive measures for deep vein thrombosis include the use of low molecular weight heparin, elastic stockings or bandages, and early mobilization.

4.7 Myocardial ischemia/infarction

The clinical manifestation occurs when an imbalance arises between the oxygen demand and myocardial oxygenation. The etiology can be categorized into two main aspects: conditions that increase oxygen demand (e.g., anemia, hypoxemia, hypotension, fever, tachycardia, surgical stress, etc.) and conditions that restrict perfusion (e.g., atherosclerosis, vasospasm, etc.). This clinical presentation is associated with significant mortality and morbidity in the postoperative period and is considered one of the primary causes of post-surgical death. The presence of risk factors such as underlying diabetes mellitus, smoking, advanced age, and family history are indications of a poor prognosis.

4.8 Arrhythmia

Arrhythmia is frequently observed in patients with a cardiac disease history. It can be classified into three main categories: tachyarrhythmias, bradyarrhythmias, and blocks. Common presenting symptoms include palpitations, chest pain, shortness of breath, hypotension, and syncope. Typically, arrhythmias are transient in nature, and it is crucial to investigate and identify the underlying causes while prioritizing hemodynamic stability.

DOI: http://dx.doi.org/10.5772/intechopen.1004839

4.9 Pneumonia

Predisposing factors for pneumonia include chronic lung diseases, smoking, and atelectasis. Patients with this condition often experience symptoms such as fever, tachypnea, and tachycardia. Aspiration pneumonia is particularly a concern for patients who undergo emergency surgery without a prior fasting period and those with intestinal obstruction. Unfortunately, the mortality rate for aspiration pneumonia exceeds 50%.

4.10 Anastomotic complications

4.10.1 Anastomotic leakage

Anastomotic leakage commonly manifests within the 5–7-day postoperative period. Clinical follow-up may reveal fever, leukocytosis, tachypnea, hypotension, localized or diffuse tenderness, ileus, tachycardia, and distension as potential findings. Early leaks are associated with high morbidity.

In large series, the intra-abdominal leak rate ranges from 1 to 5%. However, when it comes to anastomoses in the pelvis, the leak rate is higher, ranging from 5 to 15%.

4.10.2 Bleeding from the anastomotic line

Bleeding from the anastomosis line is uncommon and usually self-limiting. However, in cases where the patient has a bleeding diathesis, it is important to correct this condition. If the bleeding persists and worsens clinically, it can be managed by placing sutures near the anal canal to control the bleeding. In the case of anastomoses in the high-level region, if bleeding cannot be successfully stopped, it may be necessary to perform a relaparotomy.

4.10.3 Anastomotic stenosis/stricture

Anastomotic stricture can be caused by various factors including ischemia, anastomotic leakage, the use of narrow staplers, radiotherapy, and proximal diversion. Stenosis in the rectum can be treated by methods such as rectal examination, surgical intervention, or balloon dilatation. On the other hand, stenosis in colonic anastomoses is less common. In large series, the rate of stenosis in rectal anastomoses is reported to be around 20%, while it is lower at approximately 1–2% in colonic anastomoses.

4.11 Stoma complications

4.11.1 Stoma ischemia and necrosis

Ischemia and necrosis occur more frequently in colostomies, particularly when the left colic artery is ligated, compared to ileostomies. An ischemic stoma can be identified by its pale, edematous, or grayish blue color. Without sufficient blood flow, the ischemic stoma can progress to necrosis over time. Consequently, it is crucial to closely observe the color of the stoma during the initial 24–48 hours following the surgery. Stoma ischemia can be caused by a narrow opening in the abdominal wall or a taut stoma opening.

4.11.2 Stoma retraction

Stoma retraction refers to the protrusion of the stoma into the abdominal cavity. While it typically occurs in the early stages, it can also manifest later on. Inadequate mobilization and fixation of the colon, as well as obesity, are contributing factors to stoma retraction. In some cases, surgical revision may be necessary to address this issue.

4.11.3 Stoma prolapse

Stoma prolapse refers to the outward protrusion of the stoma from the abdominal wall. In terms of functionality, stoma prolapse does not typically pose significant implications for the patient. This complication usually arises in the later stages following the surgery. The risk of stoma prolapse is greater in ostomies created from the transverse colon, ostomies with a wide opening that is inadequately secured to the abdominal wall, patients with weak abdominal fascia, and elderly individuals. Mild cases of prolapse can often be managed through manual reduction.

4.11.4 Stoma obstruction

Stoma obstruction commonly occurs in the later stages following the surgery. In the case of ileostomies, intestinal adhesion, volvulus, and stoma stenosis are among the factors contributing to obstruction. Specifically, obstruction caused by food intake is most frequently observed during the third and sixth months following the surgery for ileostomy patients. As for colostomies, causes of obstruction can include stenosis or parastomal hernia. Additionally, tumor recurrence and hardened stool are also potential factors leading to colostomy obstruction.

4.12 Wound site infection

Infection in the surgical wound typically occurs on the third or fourth day following the operation. Clinical indications of infection encompass erythema, stiffness, edema, enlargement, and elevated temperature in the wound area. The puncture or opening of the wound may yield purulent, hemopurulent, or seropurulent discharge. If left untreated, wound infection can lead to wound dehiscence. Treatment options usually involve drainage and administration of antibiotherapy.

5. Impact of perioperative interventions on complications

The extensive research and debate surrounding the role of mechanical bowel preparation in preventing surgical site infections is an ongoing topic of interest in the medical field. However, the existing data on this subject are often conflicting, and arguments for or against bowel preparation tend to be driven by personal preference rather than strong evidence.

There are limited available data regarding the use of oral antibiotic preparation without mechanical bowel cleansing. A study published in 2017 utilized data from the American College of Surgeons National Surgical Quality Improvement Program (NSQIP) to compare different patient groups. Among the 14,080 patients included in the study, 1461 received only oral antibiotics, 9800 received mechanical bowel cleansing, and 8819 received both oral antibiotics and mechanical bowel cleansing.

When comparing the group that received oral antibiotics alone with the group that underwent mechanical bowel cleansing, several outcomes were assessed. These included surgical site infection, anastomotic leakage, postoperative ileus, and major morbidity after colorectal surgery. Interestingly, the study found that the group receiving oral antibiotics alone had decreased rates of these complications compared to the group that underwent mechanical bowel cleansing. Based on these findings, the study suggests that the addition of mechanical bowel cleansing may not be necessary in the context of oral antibiotic administration. However, it is important to note that this study is retrospective and utilized data from a national database. Therefore, it is recommended that further research, specifically randomized controlled trials, be conducted to provide a more definitive understanding of this issue.

There are several skin preparation techniques and products that exist for colorectal procedures; however, a clear consensus regarding their efficacy is currently lacking. A randomized controlled trial revealed that the utilization of chlorhexidine-alcohol, as opposed to povidone-iodine, resulted in a notable reduction of both superficial surgical site infections and deep incisional infections.

The implementation of an active heating strategy perioperatively has been demonstrated to decrease surgical site infections in patients undergoing colorectal surgery.

The PROXI study evaluated whether the administration of 80% oxygen during anesthesia in individuals undergoing abdominal surgery is effective in reducing the occurrence of surgical site infections, while ensuring that the incidence of pulmonary complications remains unaffected. Prior research has proposed that the use of 80% oxygen during surgery may decrease the likelihood of surgical wound infections, but the results have not been uniformly established. Moreover, the impact of 80% oxygen on pulmonary complications remains poorly understood.

6. The effect of post-operative interventions on complications

The incorrect administration of intravenous fluids has been identified as a contributing factor to postoperative complications. A study indicated that patients who received restricted fluids experienced earlier return of bowel function, shorter hospital stays, and lower rates of complications.

The findings of a meta-analysis of randomized controlled trials reveal that patients who were treated with the Enhanced Recovery After Surgery (ERAS) protocol, which includes fluid restriction, experienced significant benefits compared to those receiving standard postoperative care. Specifically, the patients in the ERAS group had an average shorter length of stay by 2.5 days and a 50% lower rate of postoperative morbidity.

Perioperative pain is recognized as a potent stimulus for the stress response, which can induce activation of the autonomic nervous system and subsequently lead to negative postoperative outcomes. While it remains uncertain whether inadequate pain control directly contributes to complications, many surgeons have embraced the principle of ensuring effective pain management as part of their postoperative care protocol.

According to a recently published meta-analysis, it was concluded that while there was an improvement in pain control with the use of epidurals in patients undergoing laparoscopic colectomy, there was no significant difference observed in terms of the return of bowel function or the length of hospital stay.

Postoperative recovery protocols in academic journals have predominantly integrated non-opioid-based pain regimens. Various studies have also emphasized the utilization of local blocks, such as the transversus abdominis plane (TAP) block, with the aim of enhancing pain management.

Intraoperative contamination poses a risk of infection, with wound hematoma or seroma acting as a potential trigger. A study involving 76 patients with high-risk wounds examined the impact of daily negative pressure wound dressing compared to standard wound treatment. The results revealed that patients treated with daily negative pressure wound dressing had lower rates of surgical site infection. Implementing this technique on contaminated wounds can effectively reduce the incidence of surgical site infections. It is worth noting that this approach is minimally invasive and may potentially lead to shorter hospital stays.

7. Factors affecting complications

Age is recognized as an independent risk factor for both morbidity and mortality, surpassing the impact of other comorbidities [3]. Elderly patients often face a higher degree of challenges regarding their ability to tolerate surgical procedures, surpassing those experienced by other age groups. Moreover, the elderly population encounters additional issues specific to their age group, including cognitive impairment and a potential lack of social support.

Studies have demonstrated a link between cognitive impairment and an increased need for higher levels of care in the older adult population. Specifically, it has been found that preoperative cognitive impairment, regardless of age, is associated with a higher likelihood of experiencing postoperative complications, an extended length of hospital stay, and a higher six-month mortality rate.

Frailty is a syndrome characterized by age-related declines in functional reserves across various physiological systems. The presence of negative energy and nutritional imbalances exacerbates frailty, thereby prolonging postoperative care for affected patients.

Obesity poses several challenges during surgical procedures, including increased technical complexity and potentially longer duration. Additionally, it significantly elevates the risk of developing wound site infections. A study conducted by Itani et al. explored the connection between body mass index (BMI) and antibiotic prophylaxis among patients undergoing elective colorectal surgery. The findings revealed a higher incidence of surgical site infections among patients with a BMI above 30 kg/m^2, irrespective of the type of prophylaxis employed [4]. Another study by Yamamoto et al. identified BMI as an independent risk factor for the development of anastomotic leakage [5]. However, BMI alone fails to encompass the full risk of obesity-related wound infections, leading to recent investigations into the role of waist circumference (WC) and waist-to-hip ratio (WHR) in perioperative outcomes. A prospective, multicenter, international study involving 1349 patients undergoing elective colorectal surgery was carried out to evaluate the impact of WC and WHR on surgical complications. The results demonstrated that increased WHR independently predicted intraoperative complications, medical complications, and reinterventions, whereas increased BMI was only associated with abdominal wall complications.

Minimally invasive surgery offers the advantage of reduced blood loss and a lower rate of blood transfusion compared to traditional open surgery. Research studies have consistently reported that perioperative blood transfusions can have detrimental effects on patient survival, and patients who receive transfusions are more likely to experience postoperative complications [6, 7]. It is worth noting that the

DOI: http://dx.doi.org/10.5772/intechopen.1004839

administration of allogeneic blood transfusions is also a well-known risk factor for surgical site infections.

The American Society of Anesthesiologists (ASA) classification system is utilized to evaluate and categorize patients prior to surgery. This classification helps determine the appropriate anesthetic approach and monitoring methods for each patient. Longo et al. conducted a study examining the factors contributing to early mortality and morbidity among patients undergoing colectomy. Their findings revealed that patients classified as ASA 3, 4, and 5 exhibited higher rates of early mortality and complications [8].

Previous research has established a connection between diabetes mellitus and a greater risk of experiencing complications related to surgical site infection. Specifically, inadequate glucose regulation has been linked to a heightened likelihood of early postoperative surgical site infection in individuals undergoing colorectal surgery.

The location of a tumor plays a role in the occurrence of complications. Studies have demonstrated that rectal tumors are more prone to developing anastomotic leakage when compared to tumors located in the colon.

In a study conducted by Hamabe et al., the correlation between neoadjuvant chemotherapy and anastomotic leakage was investigated. The results indicated that the risk of experiencing anastomotic leakage was 3.5 times greater in patients who received neoadjuvant chemotherapy, as determined through multivariate analysis [9].

As the size of a tumor increases, there are limitations on intrapelvic manipulation, and the process of rectal transection becomes more challenging. Consequently, tumor size has been identified as a potential risk factor for anastomotic leakage. In a study comprising 154 rectal cancer patients, findings revealed a four-fold increased risk of anastomotic leakage in tumors that were equal to or larger than 5 cm in diameter [10].

According to existing literature, it has been noted that there is a higher incidence of anastomotic leakage following colorectal surgery among male patients. This observation has been attributed to potential technical challenges arising from the narrower pelvis in male individuals.

Considerable attention has been devoted to investigating the influence of surgical volume on the occurrence of complications. The relationship between the volume of surgeons and that of the medical institutions involved may be intricately interconnected. Prior reviews and meta-analyses, which primarily focused on patients treated prior to 2000, presented conflicting findings concerning the association between hospital or surgeon volume and outcomes in rectal cancer cases. With advancements in rectal cancer resection techniques, such as total mesorectal excision, it is crucial to establish whether surgical volume has an impact on outcomes in patients treated since 2000. Through a systematic literature search and meta-analysis comprising 2845 assessed articles, only 21 satisfied the specified inclusion and exclusion criteria. The study's conclusion supports the notion that higher hospital volume among patients diagnosed since 2000 has shown a significant protective effect on outcomes for rectal cancer surgery [11].

8. Impact of complications on survival

Postoperative complications are widely recognized to have detrimental effects on both short-term quality of life and the financial burden of care. Additionally, emerging evidence suggests that these complications can also negatively influence long-term oncologic outcomes.

A conducted study by the Dutch cancer group focused on evaluating 11,000 stage-3 colorectal cancer patients within the period of 2008 to 2013. Among these patients, 4899 individuals did not receive adjuvant chemotherapy. In this group, the five-year survival rate was found to be merely 39%. However, when chemotherapy was initiated after the 12th week following surgery, the five-year survival rate witnessed a significant increase to 54%. Moreover, early initiation of chemotherapy, specifically within six weeks after surgery, resulted in a remarkable 5-year survival rate of 76%. These findings highlight the crucial impact of timely administration of adjuvant treatment on patient prognosis. Consequently, mitigating postoperative complications assumes added significance in terms of enhancing patient outcomes [12].

Complications that occur following surgery for colorectal cancer have been associated with a negative effect on survival rates. For instance, a meta-analysis examining the implications of anastomotic leakage revealed a decrease in survival rates along with an increased risk of local recurrence [13]. Similarly, another meta-analysis concentrating on patients with colorectal cancer emphasized the detrimental impact of infective complications on both disease-free survival and overall survival [14].

Postoperative complications may result in the delayed or complete cessation of chemotherapy in patients who have clear indications for systemic treatment.

Author details

Veysel Cem Ozcan
Ankara University Faculty of Medicine, Department of Surgical Oncology, Ankara, Turkey

*Address all correspondence to: dr_cemzcan@yahoo.com

References

[1] Kang JC, Chung MH, Chao PC, Yeh CC, Hsiao CW, Lee TY, et al. Hand-assisted laparoscopic colectomy vs open colectomy: A prospective randomized study. Surgical Endoscopy. 2004;**18**(4):577-581. DOI: 10.1007/s00464-003-8148-3

[2] Lindsey I, George B, Kettlewell M, Mortensen N. Randomized, double-blind, placebo-controlled trial of sildenafil (Viagra®) for erectile dysfunction after rectal excision for cancer and inflammatory bowel disease. Diseases of the Colon and Rectum. 2002;**45**(6):727-732. DOI: 10.1007/s10350-004-6287-9

[3] Jafari MD, Jafari F, Halabi WJ, Nguyen VQ, Pigazzi A, Carmichael JC, et al. Colorectal cancer resections in the aging US population: A trend toward decreasing rates and improved outcomes. JAMA Surgery. 2014;**149**(6):557-564. DOI: 10.1001/jamasurg.2013.4930

[4] Itani KM, Jensen EH, Finn TS, Tomassini JE, Abramson MA. Effect of body mass index and ertapenem versus cefotetan prophylaxis on surgical site infection in elective colorectal surgery. Surgical Infections. 2008;**9**(2):131-137. DOI: 10.1089/sur.2007.034

[5] Yamamoto S, Fujita S, Akasu T, Inada R, Moriya Y, Yamamoto S. Risk factors for anastomotic leakage after laparoscopic surgery for rectal cancer using a stapling technique. Surgical Laparoscopy, Endoscopy & Percutaneous Techniques. 2012;**22**(3):239-243. DOI: 10.1097/SLE.0b013e31824fbb56

[6] Patel SV, Brennan KE, Nanji S, Karim S, Merchant S, Booth CM. Peri-operative blood transfusion for resected colon cancer: Practice patterns and outcomes in a population-based study. Cancer Epidemiology. 2017;**51**:35-40. DOI: 10.1016/j.canep.2017.10.006

[7] Mazzeffi M, Tanaka K, Galvagno S. Red blood cell transfusion and surgical site infection after colon resection surgery: A cohort study. Anesthesia and Analgesia. 2017;**125**(4):1316-1321. DOI: 10.1213/ANE.0000000000002099

[8] Longo WE, Virgo KS, Johnson FE, Oprian CA, Vernava AM, Wade TP, et al. Risk factors for morbidity and mortality after colectomy for colon cancer. Diseases of the Colon and Rectum. 2000;**43**(1):83-91. DOI: 10.1007/BF02237249

[9] Hamabe A, Ito M, Nishigori H, Nishizawa Y, Sasaki T. Preventive effect of diverting stoma on anastomotic leakage after laparoscopic low anterior resection with double stapling technique reconstruction applied based on risk stratification. Asian Journal of Endoscopic Surgery. 2018;**11**(3):220-226. DOI: 10.1111/ases.12439

[10] Kawada K, Hasegawa S, Hida K, Hirai K, Okoshi K, Nomura A, et al. Risk factors for anastomotic leakage after laparoscopic low anterior resection with DST anastomosis. Surgical Endoscopy. 2014;**28**(10):2988-2995. DOI: 10.1007/s00464-014-3564-0

[11] Chioreso C, Del Vecchio N, Schweizer ML, Schlichting J, Gribovskaja-Rupp I, Charlton ME. Association between hospital and surgeon volume and rectal cancer surgery outcomes in patients with rectal cancer treated since 2000: Systematic literature review and meta-analysis. Diseases of the Colon and Rectum. 2018;**61**(11):1320-1332. DOI: 10.1097/DCR.0000000000001198

[12] Bos AC, van Erning FN, van Gestel YR, Creemers GJ, Punt CJ, van Oijen MG, et al. Timing of adjuvant chemotherapy and its relation to survival among patients with stage III colon cancer. European Journal of Cancer. 2015;**51**(17):2553-2561. DOI: 10.1016/j.ejca.2015.08.016

[13] Mirnezami A, Mirnezami R, Chandrakumaran K, Sasapu K, Sagar P, Finan P. Increased local recurrence and reduced survival from colorectal cancer following anastomotic leak: Systematic review and meta-analysis. Annals of Surgery. 2011;**253**(5):890-899. DOI: 10.1097/SLA.0b013e3182128929

[14] Pucher PH, Aggarwal R, Qurashi M, Darzi A. Meta-analysis of the effect of postoperative in-hospital morbidity on long-term patient survival. The British Journal of Surgery. 2014;**101**(12):1499-1508. DOI: 10.1002/bjs.9615

Chapter 7

IP6 + Ins in the Treatment of Colon Cancer Patients during Chemotherapy: Observational Clinical Study

Nikica Druzijanic, Ana Druzijanic and Ivana Vucenik

Abstract

Although multiple health-beneficial effects have been related to inositol hexaphosphate (IP6), the most striking is its anticancer effect. This natural, highly phosphorylated carbohydrate and its parent compound, myo-inositol (Ins), are abundantly present in plants, but also in mammalian cells, where they regulate important cellular functions. IP6 reduces proliferation and induces apoptosis and differentiation of malignant cells, enhances immunity, and affects several critical molecular targets. The best results were obtained from the combination of IP6 + Ins. Available as a dietary supplement, IP6 + Ins can enhance the anticancer effect of conventional chemotherapy, and improve quality of life in cancer patients, reducing burden of chemotherapy. Here we present the first, but encouraging, clinical observational study with IP6 and Ins in colon cancer patients during chemotherapy. These results were the basis for several randomized controlled trials organized later. We hope that more clinical trials and mechanistic studies would follow to clarify these intriguing findings.

Keywords: cancer prevention and treatment, phytic acid, molecular targets, colon cancer, clinical study

1. Introduction

Cancer is still rapidly growing, representing one of the major global health problems. Today we know that more than one-half of cancer cases and deaths are potentially preventable by modifications of major risk factors, such as smoking, unhealthy diet, consumption of alcohol, physical inactivity, and overweight and obesity [1]. By increasing vegetable intake, maintaining the optimum body weight and regular physical activity, it has been shown that 30–40% of cancers could be prevented [2, 3], even more, if we can apply the knowledge about cancer prevention, the obstacles are socio-economic reasons.

Globally, colorectal cancer (CRC) is the third most common cancer [4]. It also represents the second leading cause of death related to cancer [4]. It was projected that over 1.9 million new CRC cases and 930,000 deaths will happen in 2020. Estimated to GLOBOCAN, by 2040 there will be 3.2 million new cases of CRC and 1.6 million deaths [4].

However, interestingly, this highly frequent cancer worldwide is largely preventable through changes in modifiable risk factors. Since diet has an important role in the etiology of CRC [4, 5], the use of natural products, that are well tolerated, have been suggested for the prevention and treatment of CRC.

IP6 (*myo*-inositol hexaphosphate, $InsP_6$, known also as phytic acid) and its parent compound *myo*-inositol (Ins) are both found in plants [6–8]. Because of its unique structure, IP6 is known and accepted as a strong antioxidant [9]. However, not only in plants, but almost all mammalian cells contain IP6 and lower inositol phosphates. These molecules have essential roles in regulating vital cellular functions and activities, energy metabolism, and signal transduction [10–12].

Here we give a brief overview of the anticancer potential of IP6, and then present the first data in a clinical setting, in patients with colon cancer during chemotherapy. This observational study provided a great basis for later clinical trials.

2. Anticancer potential of IP6

2.1 Cancer preventive and therapeutic activities

The first preclinical studies showing anticancer potential of IP6 in colon cancer were conducted by Shamsuddin *et al.* [13–15]. IP6 was given in drinking water to experimental animals and was able to prevent colon cancer using different animal models (rats and mice) and even when using different carcinogens (1,2-dimethylhydrazine and azoxymethane) [13–21]. IP6 was potent and effective in inhibiting colon cancer in a dose-dependent manner given either before or after carcinogen administration. However, extremely exciting was the finding that IP6 was able to reduce the development of large intestinal cancer even when given after carcinogen administration. This ability of IP6 to significantly lower tumor number and size even 5 months after administration, had suggested its potential use of IP6 as a therapeutic agent [15]. Furthermore, in these first experimental studies with IP6 in colon cancer, other investigators (Drs. Pretlow and Reddy) demonstrated a decreased incidence of aberrant crypts, the parameter that has been often utilized as an intermediate biomarker for colon cancer at that time [18, 19]. A broad-spectrum anticancer activity was shown against cancers of different cells and different tissue systems, where IP6 inhibited growth of malignant cells, induced differentiation in K-562 hematopoietic cells [22], HT-29 cells human colon carcinoma [23, 24], prostate, breast, and rhabdomyosarcoma cancer cells [25] *in vitro*. Additionally, *in vivo* experiments showed cancer preventive and protective effects of IP6 in breast cancer [25], skin cancer [26, 27], and prostate cancer [28].

The therapeutic properties of IP6 were shown in the FSA-1 mouse model of transplantable and metastatic fibrosarcoma [29], in human rhabdomyosarcoma [30], and experimental hepatoma model [31]. In a human rhabdomyosarcoma (RD) animal model, RD cells were transplanted in nude mice [30], and the efficacy of IP6 was tested on the tumor-forming capacity of RD cells during the peritumoral treatment with IP6, initiated 2 days after subcutaneous injection of RD cells. In this model, IP6 was able to suppress tumor growth by 25–49-fold [30]. Furthermore, IP6 was also potent to inhibit experimental hepatoma [31, 32], when the efficacy of IP6 was tested on tumorigenicity and on tumor regression. While a single treatment of HepG2 cells *in vitro* by IP6 resulted in a complete loss of their ability to form tumors when inoculated subcutaneously in nude mice [31], a dramatic regression of liver cancers was demonstrated when tumors were treated directly with IP6 [31].

2.2 Possible mechanisms

It has been hypothesized and then shown in many experimental models that Ins potentiates both the antiproliferative and antineoplastic effects of IP6 *in vivo* in colon, mammary cancer, and in metastatic lung cancer model [25]. In a series of preclinical experiments Dr. Song Yang was studying colon cancer and its metastasis to the liver [33–35], also demonstrating that Ins potentiates the anticancer effect of IP6. They showed that when combining IP6 and Ins, the survival of experimental animals was improved, while the tumor mass and liver metastasis were decreased. Because metastasis is a primary cause of death in colon cancer patients, and the liver is the most common site, the work of Dr. Song Yang and his group is very important [33–35].

Today we better understand the role of IP6, Ins and inositol phosphates, and their involvement in multiple biochemical pathways and cellular interactions. We know that almost all animal cells contain inositol phosphates that affect and regulate multiple cell functions, signal transduction, and energy metabolism. The specific role of IP6 among these multiple signaling pathways is very complex and still needs to be studied in the future. Briefly, IP6 can modulate cellular response at the level of receptor binding, can affect few critical molecular targets in the cell cycle (p27, pRB phosphorylation), signal transduction (PI3K, PKC/RAS/ERK, Akt, ERK), and inflammation (NF-κB). Several broad and extensive reviews of the anticancer activity of IP6 and Ins have been published [25, 36–39]. In this report, we mentioned briefly some of the most important cellular mechanisms and molecular interaction of IP6 and would like to focus on those important in colon cancer science and clinical applications.

2.3 IP6 in colon cancer

Regarding the anticancer effect of IP6 in colon cancer, a wide range of results starting from the initial aberrant crypt foci, an early biomarker of colon carcinogenesis [25] to the novel regulation of microRNA-155 and its related gene expression [40] have been shown. Very novel are mechanisms related to the anti-metastatic effects of IP6 and Ins in a liver metastasis model of colorectal cancer in BALB/c mice, that involve the changing expression of the extracellular matrix proteins collagen IV, fibronectin, and laminin, the adhesion factor receptor integrin-β1, the proteolytic enzyme matrix metalloproteinase 9, and the angiogenic factors vascular endothelial growth factor, basic fibroblast growth factor, and transforming growth factor beta in the tumor metastasis microenvironment [33]. Trying to better understand the mechanism of inhibiting tumor progression and liver metastasis of colorectal cancer, Dr. Song's team utilized an orthotopic transplantation model of colorectal cancer [34] and monitored the expression of genes related to the Wnt/β-catenin in this model. Their results of real-time PCR and Western blot indicated that mRNA and protein expressions of β-catenin, Wnt10b, Tcf7, and c-Myc were significantly lower in IP6 + Ins group [34].

In addition to its role and effects on tumor, IP6 can act on host's immune system. It was shown that IP6 can boost natural killer cell (NK) activity [41, 42].

Interestingly, the inverse relationship between NK activity and tumor incidence was shown. An increase in cancer incidence is associated with a decreased NK cell activity, while increased NK activity, induced by IP6 is related to decreased tumor incidence.

Furthermore, the sensitivity and selectivity of IP6 were shown, with ability to target malignant cells without affecting normal cells and tissues [25]. Also, IP6 was able to acts synergistically with standard chemotherapeutics and to overcome the acquired drug resistance [25].

3. IP6 + Ins in the treatment of colon cancer patients during chemotherapy: observational clinical study

IP6 + Ins has been available as a supplement for over 20 years. Both IP6 and Ins met specifications of the FDA, and both have been given GRAS (Generally Recognized As Safe) status. As a part of regular diet, both IP6 and Ins have very low toxicity and therefore can be used to enhance the anticancer effect of conventional chemotherapy with almost no, or very few side effects. Here we present observational clinical study of colon cancer patients who were taking IP6 + Ins supplement during chemotherapy. This study has never been published but served as a basis for several, organized clinical studies.

3.1 Methods

In the period from 2000 to 2004, 22 patients with colon cancer stage Dukes B and higher, treated at the University Hospital Split, Croatia were included in the study. All patients were treated with postoperative chemotherapy. Data from preoperative and postoperative evaluation, which included abdominal CT and ultrasound, lung X-ray, complete blood count with differentials, biochemical laboratory tests, tumor markers: CEA, CA 19–9, and pathohistological findings were included in this study. Chemotherapy was administered according to the "Mayo Clinic" protocol, 5 days/6 weeks, with 5-FU 425 mg/m^2, and Leucovorine 20 mg/m^2. Radiotherapy was administered in 25 cycles of 2 Gy. IP6 + Ins regimen during chemotherapy was 4 capsules (2040 mg) thrice daily, 30 minutes before meals. Following chemotherapy, the IP6 + Ins regimen was 2 capsules (1020 mg), thrice daily, before meals. Chemotherapy-related side-effects were monitored in all patients, namely: drop in leukocyte and platelet counts, nausea, vomiting, stomatitis, fever, diarrhea, alopecia, and neurological disorders (paraesthesia).

Statistical analysis was performed using t-test, Friedman's test for finding differences in treatments across multiple attempts, and repeated measures ANOVA. p-value <0.05 was considered significant.

3.2 Results

Out of 22 participants, 16 were males. The average age for male participants was 64 years (41–71), and for females 66 years (54–70). Colon cancer was classified as Dukes B in 8, Dukes C in 10, and Dukes D in 4 participants. The right hemicolectomy was performed in 3 patients, sub-total colectomy in 3, anterior resection of rectum in 12, and amputation of rectum in 4 patients. Laboratory results and their comparison during chemotherapy, at the middle and the end of chemotherapy are shown in

	Middle of the chemotherapy	End of the chemotherapy	p-value
Hematocrit (L/L)	0.33	0.33	0.15
Platelets (× 10^9/L)	240	231	0.37
AST (U/L)	17.9	19.6	0.47
Creatinine (µmol/L)	94.1	95.5	0.50
BUN (mmol/L)	5.9	6.0	0.68
Glucose (mmol/L)	5.6	5.7	0.58
CEA (ng/mL)	7.3	7.5	0.84
CA 19–9 (U/mL)	16.8	19.4	0.16

Table 1.
Comparison of the laboratory results during chemotherapy and IP6 + Ins.

Table 1. There were no significant changes in these values during chemotherapy in patients who were receiving IP6 + Ins (t-test).

Table 2 shows comparison of the mean blood counts (erythrocytes, leukocytes, platelets) at the beginning of chemotherapy, during, and at the end of chemotherapy, evaluated by the Friedman's test. It is known that chemotherapy can damage bone marrow and produce low counts of erythrocytes, leukocytes, and platelets, causing anemia, septicemia, and bleeding. Therefore, if the blood cell levels are too low, the next treatment might be put off until these levels recover: this is known as "chemo break". Although there were changes in blood counts during chemotherapy, these levels were never so low that threatened patients' lives, and chemotherapy was never interrupted (no need for "chemo break").

Thrombocytopenia and neutropenia are usual side effects of chemotherapy. However, **Figures 1** and **2** demonstrate that in two patients (Cases 1 and 2), as representatives of the group, during chemotherapy white blood cell counts (leukocytes) and platelet counts did not drop when IP6 + Ins were given to the patients, as also shown in **Table 2**.

Metastases in colorectal cancer are most commonly found in the liver and lungs. **Figure 3** shows CT scan of lung metastases in a Duke's D colon cancer patient in 2 years, indicating very slow progression of the existing and the absence of any new metastatic lesions.

In the observed period, 3 patients died. All other patients received full dose of chemotherapy and radiotherapy, without breaks ("chemo break").

3.3 Discussion

Because preclinical and encouraging clinical data suggest that IP6 and Ins are promising in prevention of cancer and as adjuvant therapy, more controlled clinical trials are needed and encouraged. Particularly, because the rising incidence and mortality for some cancers are of concern, and CRC is on the rise in USA among young people, despite the decrease in overall cancer frequency and death rate, that overall are encouraging. Currently, CRC is the fourth most common cancer in the United States. It was predicted that in 2023, approximately 153,020 individuals will be diagnosed with CRC and 52,550 will die from the disease [4]. However, among these, about 20,000 cases and 3750 deaths are expected in individuals younger than 50 years, which is concerning and alarming [4].

Erythrocytes (E) (× 10^{12}/L)				Leukocytes (L) (× 10^{9}/L)				Platelets (P) (× 10^{9}/L)			
E0	E1	E2	p-value	L0	L1	L2	p-value	P0	P1	P3	p-value
4.3	4.0	3.9	0.0007	7.3	5.5	4.7	0.000	281	240	230	0.00008

0 = beginning of chemotherapy; 1 = middle of chemotherapy; 2 = end of chemotherapy.

Table 2.
Changes in blood count values in patients on chemotherapy and IP6 + Ins.

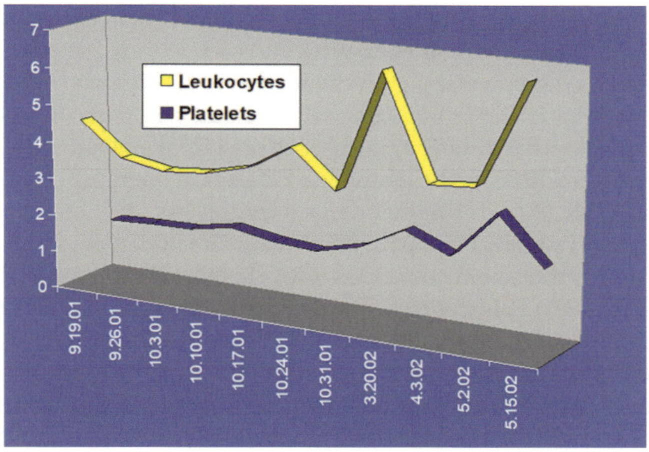

Figure 1.
Leucocytes and platelet counts shown during chemotherapy (Case 1).

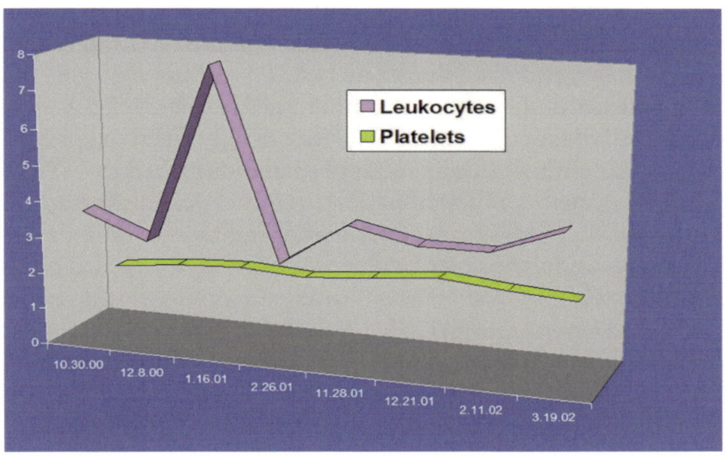

Figure 2.
Leucocytes and platelet counts shown during chemotherapy (Case 2).

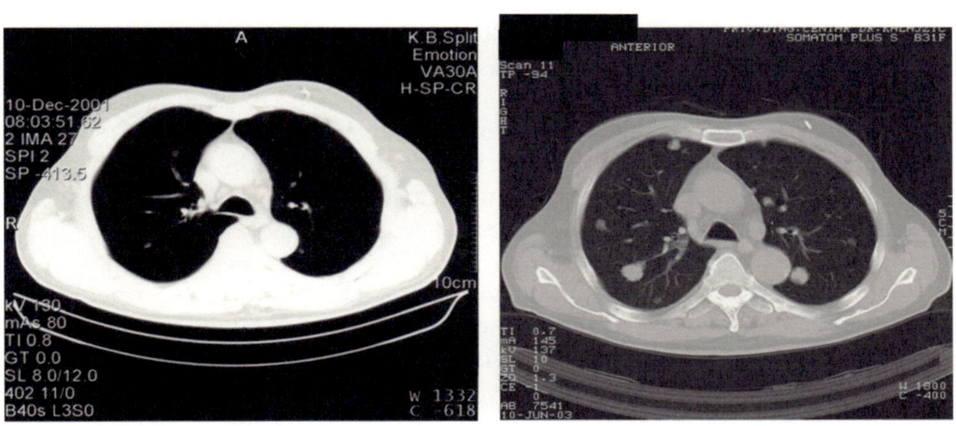

Figure 3.
Lung metastases in a Duke's D colon cancer patient, showing CT scan in 2001 (left) and in 2003 (right).

During chemotherapy, in most patients, some anomalies in their complete blood count, primarily in the number of leukocytes and platelets are happening. Studies also have associated chemotherapy with the increased risk of gastrointestinal, hematologic, and cardiac toxicities in patients with colon cancer, with the most common hematological adverse effect being agranulocytosis [43]. However, when IP6 + Ins was given in combination with chemotherapy, side effects of chemotherapy were reduced and patients were able to perform their daily activities [44, 45]. In a case study of lung cancer, the long-term survival of a patient with advanced non-small cell lung cancer treated with IP_6 + Ins treatment combined with chemo-radiotherapy was reported [46]. In a phase I clinical study with Ins, it was shown that Ins was safe and well tolerated [47]. When IP6 was combined with beta-(1,3)/(1,6) D-glucan, the favorable and beneficial effect on hematopoiesis in the treatment of patients with advanced malignancies receiving chemotherapy was demonstrated [48]. The combination of IP6 and Ins diminished the negative side effects of chemotherapy and preserved quality of life in breast cancer patients in a small prospective, randomized, pilot clinical study [44]. In a double-blind, randomized controlled trial (RCT) in women with ductal breast cancer, topical IP6 treatment was effective and safe in preventing and/or mitigating chemotherapy-induced side effects and was able to preserve quality of life [49]. To further identify the clinical evidence of the effectiveness of IP6 and Ins on the quality of life in cancer patients, and to demonstrate that IP6 and Ins were able to improve the quality of life in patients undergoing chemotherapy due to breast cancer, a literature search was conducted to identify clinical evidence of the effectiveness of IP6 and Ins on the quality of life in cancer patient and indeed demonstrated that IP6 and Ins were effective in improving quality of life of patients receiving chemotherapy due to breast cancer [50]. In a cohort of breast cancer patients, a combined oral-local treatment with IP6 and Ins was conducted, with oral myo-inositol + IP6 local application. This combined treatment with IP6 and Ins was also able to improve local symptoms and quality-of-life-related symptoms [51].

A remarkable case report on melanoma was presented by Khurana *et al.* [52]. The patient was with metastatic melanoma and declined traditional therapy. Instead, he decided to try the IP6 + Ins supplement only. To their surprise, the patient achieved a complete remission and remains in remission 3 years later. This might indicate a new pathway for IP6 in clinical practice - immunotherapy, a potential for immune-stimulating effects of IP6 and Ins in patients with metastatic melanoma could be explored.

In this pilot clinical observational study, a group of patients with multiple liver and lung metastases, IP6 + Ins was given as an adjuvant to chemotherapy according to Mayo protocol. Our results showed that no patient had to discontinue chemotherapy due to abnormality of hematological and/or biochemical parameters. Three patients died during the observed period. The first patient died 11 months after operation due to myocardial infarction, other two patients died 30 and 33 months after the surgery, respectively, due to dissemination of colorectal cancer. All deceased patients had colorectal cancer classified as Dukes D.

This study indicated that IP6 and Ins contributed to the anticancer effect of chemotherapy and improved the quality of life. This was a non-randomized clinical trial, which did not allow us to compare the outcome with patients without IP6 and Ins treatment. Side-effects were monitored by clinical observation, while standardized questionnaires were not used. However, based on this initial clinical observational study, a first prospective, randomized, pilot clinical study with IP6 + Ins was organized and conducted [44].

4. Conclusion

Available as dietary supplements, both with a GRAS status, IP6 and Ins have been in clinical practice for over 20 years. From many case reports, some anecdotal evidence, and few small clinical studies, the enhanced antitumor activity with improved quality of life by IP6, Ins, and their combination with reduced tumor growth rate and in some cases, even a regression of primary lesions, was reported.

Judged by multiple experimental and clinical data, it has been shown that IP6 + Ins can be a new option for cancer prevention, but also for cancer treatment, and always with ability to reduce the chemotherapy-induced side-effects. However, still more experimental data and a more controlled clinical study are needed to evaluate the antitumoral effect of IP6 + Inositol in cancer prevention and treatment and to better understand the mode of its action.

Conflicts of interest

All authors declare that there is no conflict of interest regarding the publication of this manuscript and that we have no financial interests in any commercial sources of inositol, IP6, or other inositol phosphates.

Author details

Nikica Druzijanic[1], Ana Druzijanic[2] and Ivana Vucenik[3,4]*

1 Department of Surgery, School of Medicine, University of Split, Split, Croatia

2 School of Medicine, Dental Medicine, Department of Oral Medicine and Periodontology, University of Split, Split, Croatia

3 Department of Medical and Research Technology, University of Maryland School of Medicine, Baltimore, USA

4 Department of Pathology, University of Maryland School of Medicine, Baltimore, USA

*Address all correspondence to: ivucenik@som.umaryland.edu

References

[1] Islami F, Goding Sauer A, Miller KD, Siegel RL, Fedewa SA, Jacobs EJ, et al. Proportion and number of cancer cases and deaths attributable to potentially modifiable risk factors in the United States. CA: A Cancer Journal for Clinicians. 2018;**68**:31-54

[2] Doll R, Peto R. The causes of cancer: Quantitative estimates of avoidable risks of cancer in the United States today. JNCI. 1981;**66**:1191-1308

[3] World Cancer Research Fund/ American Institute for Cancer Research. Diet, Nutrition, Physical Activity and Cancer: A Global Perspective. 2018

[4] Morgan E, Arnold M, Gini A, Lorenzoni V, Cabasag CJ, Laversanne M, et al. Global burden of colorectal cancer in 2020 and 2040; Incidence and mortality estimated from GLOBOCAN. Gut. 2023;**72**:338-344

[5] Rajamanickam S, Agarwal R. Natural products and colon cancer: Current status and future prospects. Drug Development Research. 2008;**69**:460-471

[6] Harland BF, Oberleas D. Phytate in foods. World Review of Nutrition and Dietetics. 1987;**52**:235-259

[7] Reddy NR, Sathe SK, Salunke DK. Phytates in legumes and cereals. Advances in Food Research. 1982;**28**:1-89

[8] Schlemmer U, Frølich RM, Prieto RM, Grases F. Phytate in foods and significance for humans: Food sources, intake, processing, bioavailability, protective role and analysis. Molecular Nutrition & Food Research. 2009;**53**(Suppl. 2):S330-S375

[9] Graf E, Eaton JW. Antioxidant functions of phytic acid. Free Radical Biology & Medicine. 1990;**8**:61-69

[10] Berridge MJ, Irvine RF. Inositol phosphates and cell signalling. Nature. 1989;**341**:197-220

[11] Shamsuddin AK, Bose S. IP6 (inositol hexaphosphate) as a signaling molecule. Current Signal Transduction Therapy. 2012;**7**:289-304

[12] Thomas MP, Mills SJ, Potter BV. The "other" inositols and their phosphates: Synthesis, biology, and medicine (with recent advances in myo-inositol chemistry). Angewandte Chemie (International Ed. in English). 2016;**55**:1614-1650

[13] Shamsuddin AM, Elsayed A, Ullah A. Suppression of large intestinal cancer in F344 rats by inositol hexaphosphate. Carcinogenesis. 1988;**9**:577-580

[14] Shamsuddin AM, Ullah A, Chakravarthy A. Inositol and inositol hexaphosphate suppress cell proliferation and tumor formation in CD-1 mice. Carcinogenesis. 1989;**10**:1461-1463

[15] Shamsuddin AM, Ullah A. Inositol hexaphosphate inhibits large intestinal cancer in F344 rats 5 months after induction by azoxymethane. Carcinogenesis. 1989;**10**:625-626

[16] Ullah A, Shamsuddin AM. Dose-dependent inhibition of large intestinal cancer by inositol hexaphosphate in F344 rats. Carcinogenesis. 1990;**11**:2219-2222

[17] Shivapurkar N, Tang ZC, Frost A, Alabaster O. A rapid dual organ rat carcinogenesis bioassay for evaluating the chemoprevention of breast and colon cancer. Cancer Letters. 1996;**100**:169-179

[18] Pretlow TP, O'Riordan MA, Somich GA, Amini SB, Pretlow TG.

Aberrant crypts correlate with tumor incidence in F344 rats treated with azoxymethane and phytate. Carcinogenesis. 1992;**13**:1509-1512

[19] Challa A, Rao DR, Reddy BS. Interactive suppression of aberrant crypt foci induced by azoxymethane in rat colon by phytic acid and green tea. Carcinogenesis. 1997;**18**:2023-2026

[20] Jenab M, Thompson LU. Phytic acid in wheat bran affects cell morphology, differentiation and apoptosis. Carcinogenesis. 2000;**21**:1547-1552

[21] Thompson LU, Zhang L. Phytic acid and minerals: Effect of early markers of risk for mammary and colon carcinogenesis. Carcinogenesis. 1991;**12**:2041-2045

[22] Deliliers LG, Servida G, Fracchiolla NS, Ricci C, Borsotti C, Colombo G, et al. Effects of inositol hexaphosphate (IP_6) on human normal and leukaemic hematopoietic cells. British Journal of Haematology. 2002;**117**:577-587

[23] Sakamoto K, Venkatraman G, Shamsuddin AM. Growth inhibition and differentiation of HT-29 cells in vitro by inositol hexaphosphate (phytic acid). Carcinogenesis. 1993;**14**:1815-1819

[24] Yang G-Y, Shamsuddin AM. IP_6-induced growth inhibition and differentiation of HT-29 human colon cancer cells: Involvement of intracellular inositol phosphates. Anticancer Research. 1995;**15**:2479-2488

[25] Vucenik I, Shamsuddin AM. Protection against cancer by dietary IP_6 and inositol. Nutrition and Cancer. 2006;**55**:109-125

[26] Williams KA, Kolappaswamy K, DeTolla LJ, Vucenik I. Protective effect of inositol hexaphosphate against UVB damage in HaCaT cells and skin carcinogenesis in SKH1 hairless mice. Comparative Medicine. 2011;**61**:39-44

[27] Kolappaswamy K, Williams KA, Benazzi C, Sarli G, McLeod CG, Vucenik I, et al. Effect of inositol hexaphosphate on UVB-induced skin tumor development in SKH1 hairless mice. Comparative Medicine. 2009;**59**:147-152

[28] Singh PR, Sharma G, Mallikarjuna GU, Dhanalakshmi S, Aragwal C, Agrwal R. In vivo suppression of hormone-refractory prostate cancer growth by inositol hexaphosphate: Induction of insulin-like growth factor binding protein-3 and inhibition of vascular endothelial growth factor. Clinical Cancer Research. 2004;**10**:244-250

[29] Vucenik I, Tomazic VJ, Fabian D, Shamsuddin AM. Antitumor activity of phytic acid (inositol hexaphosphate) in murine transplanted and metastatic fibrosarcoma, a pilot study. Cancer Letters. 1992;**65**:9-13

[30] Vucenik I, Kalebic T, Tantivejkul K, Shamsuddin AM. Novel anticancer function of inositol hexaphosphate (IP_6): Inhibition of human rhabdomyosarcoma in vitro and in vivo. Anticancer Research. 1998;**18**:1377-1384

[31] Vucenik I, Zhang ZS, Shamsuddin AM. IP_6 in treatment of liver cancer. II. Intra-tumoral injection of IP_6 regresses pre-existing human liver cancer xenotransplanted in nude mice. Anticancer Research. 1998;**18**:4091-4096

[32] Vucenik I, Tantivejkul K, Zhang ZS, Cole KE, Saied I, Shamsuddin AM. IP_6 treatment of liver cancer. I. IP_6 inhibits growth and reverses transformed phenotype in HepG2 human liver

cancer cell line. Anticancer Research. 1998;**18**:4083-4090

[33] Fu M, Song Y, Wen Z, Lu X, Cui L. Inositol Hexaphosphate and inositol inhibit colorectal cancer metastasis to the liver in BALB/c mice. Nutrients. 2016;**8**(5):286

[34] Liu X, Liu C, Chen C, Sun W, Ci Y, Li Q, et al. Combination of inositol hexaphosphate and inositol inhibits liver metastasis of colorectal cancer in mice through the Wnt/β-catenin pathway. Oncotargets and Therapy. 2020;**13**:3223-3235

[35] Li C, Ci Y, Liu X, Chen C, Liu C, Li X, et al. Inositol hexakisphosphate and inositol enhance the inhibition of colorectal cancer growth and liver metastasis by capecitabine in a mouse model. Nutrition and Cancer. 2021;**73**(11-12):2306-2314

[36] Brehm MA, Windhorst S. New options of cancer treatment employing InsP6. Biochemical Pharmacology. 2019;**163**:206-214

[37] Bizzarri M, Dinicola S, Bevilacqua A, Cucina A. Broad spectrum anticancer activity of myo-inositol and inositol hexakisphosphate. International Journal of Endocrinology. 2016;**2016**:5616807

[38] Vucenik I, Stains J. Cancer preventive and therapeutic properties of IP_6: Efficacy and mechanisms. Periodicum Biologorum. 2010;**112**:451-458

[39] Vucenik I. Anticancer properties of inositol hexaphosphate and inositol: An overview. Journal of Nutritional Science and Vitaminology (Tokyo). 2019;**65**(Supplement):S18-S22

[40] Kapral M, Wawszczyk J, Węglarz L. Regulation of microRNA-155 and its related genes expression by inositol hexaphosphate in colon cancer cells. Molecules. 2019;**24**(22):4153

[41] Baten A, Ullah A, Tomazic VJ, Shamsuddin AM. Inositol-phosphate-induced enhancement of natural killer cell activity correlates with tumor suppression. Carcinogenesis. 1989;**10**:1595-1598

[42] Zhang Z, Song Y, Wang X-L. Inositol hexaphosphate-induced enhancement of natural killer cell activity correlates with suppression of colon carcinogenesis in rats. World Journal of Gastroenterology. 2005;**11**:5044-5046

[43] Hu C-Y, Chan W, Delclos GP, Du XL. Adjuvant chemotherapy and risk of gastrointestinal, hematologic, and cardiac toxicities in elderly patients with stage III colon cancer. American Journal of Clinical Oncology. 2012;**35**:228-236

[44] Bačić I, Družijanić N, Karlo R, Škifić I, Jagić S. Efficacy of IP_6 + inositol in the treatment of breast cancer patients receiving chemotherapy: Prospective, randomized, pilot clinical study. Journal of Experimental & Clinical Cancer Research. 2010;**29**(1):12

[45] Družijanić N, Juričić J, Perko Z, Kraljević D. IP_6 + inositol as adjuvant to chemotherapy of colon cancer: Our clinical experience. Anticancer Research. 2004;**24**:3474

[46] Sakamoto K. Long-term survival of a patient with advanced non-small cell lung cancer treated with inositol Hexaphosphate (IP_6) plus inositol treatment combined with chemo-radiotherapy. Report of case. Anticancer Research. 2004;**24**:3618

[47] Lam S, McWilliams A, LeRiche J, MacAulay C, Wattenberg L, Szabo E. A phase I study of myo-inositol for lung cancer chemoprevention. Cancer

Epidemiology, Biomarkers & Prevention. 2006;**15**:1526-1531

[48] Weitberg AB. A phase I/II trial of beta-(1,3)/(1,6) D-glucan in the treatment of patients with advanced malignancies receiving chemotherapy. Journal of Experimental & Clinical Cancer Research. 2008;**27**:40

[49] Proietti S, Pasta V, Cucina A, Aragona C, Palimbi E, Vucenik I, et al. Inositol hexaphosphate (InsP6) as an effective topical treatment for patients receiving chemotherapy after surgery. European Review for Medical and Pharmacological Sciences. 2017;**21**(Suppl. 2):43-50

[50] Verna R, Guiliani A, Todde V, Minini M, Unfer V. Reduced burden of chemotherapy side-effects in patients receiving inositol hexakisphosphate alone or in association with myo-inositol. Journal of Cancer Research and Therapeutics. 2018;**3**:1-5

[51] Amabile ML, De Luca A, Tripodi D, D'Alberti E. Effects of inositol hexaphosphate and myoinositol administration in breast cancer patients during adjuvant chemotherapy. Journal of Personalized Medicine. 2021;**11**(8):756

[52] Khurana S, Baldeo C, Joseph RW. Inositol hexaphosphate plus inositol induced complete remission in stage IV melanoma: A case report. Melanoma Research. 2019;**2019**(29):322-324

Chapter 8

Revealing Colon Cancer Resistance with Identification of Glutamate Metabolites by Proton MR Spectroscopy In Vivo and the Molecular Mechanism

Qi Xie, Yi-Ming Yang, Min-Yi Wu, Xi-Yan Shao, Gui-Qin Wang and Jing Zhang

Abstract

This study aimed to investigate the ability of 1H-MRS to evaluate drug-resistant colon cancer in vivo. Xenograft tumour mouse models were generated by parental SW480 cells (5-FU-responsive) or SW480/5-FU cells (5-FU-resistant). After 1H-MRS was performed on these Xenograft tumour mouse models, the tumour lesions were resected for the in vitro assessment of the expression of drug resistance-related proteins and glutathione metabolism-related enzymes. The tumours from SW480/5-FU mice showed significantly higher levels of choline, Glx1, and Glx2 detected by 1H-MRS than the tumours from SW480 mice ($P < 0.05$). The SW480/5-FU tumours also showed higher expression of glutathione metabolism-related enzymes ($P < 0.05$). The 1H-MRS-detected metabolites showed positive correlations with the expression levels of drug resistance-related proteins and glutathione metabolism-related enzymes. Glx1 and Glx2 metabolites detected in vivo by 1H-MRS may be biomarkers of 5-FU drug resistance in colon cancer.

Keywords: proton magnetic resonance spectroscopy (1H-MRS), glutathione, human colon cancer, tumour xenograft model, multiple drug resistance

1. Introduction

The most common treatment for patients with advanced colorectal cancer (CRC) is palliative chemotherapy with a 5-fluorouracil (5-FU)-based regimen [1]. Unfortunately, the progression-free survival period is only 8.7–12.3 months [2]. Multidrug resistance (MDR) occurs frequently and remains the major obstacle in CRC treatment [2–4].

For patients with CRC, knowledge of the drug resistance status of their tumour(s) is very important because this information will serve as the basis for the therapeutic strategy and adjusting this strategy as the treatment progresses. At present, drug sensitivity/resistance testing relies on in vitro assays [5]. The tumour is a heterogeneous and pleomorphic cell group with irregular differentiation. Because a biopsy is required to obtain tumour tissue for testing via the in vitro method, the drug resistance status detected is representative of only the biopsy area, and that of the remaining tumour in situ is unknown. The invasive biopsy procedure itself is a major drawback. Moreover, the time needed for obtaining a clinical sample and laboratory testing is long. Undoubtedly, an in vivo method that will accurately and conveniently evaluate the drug resistance status of a tumour is urgently needed.

Studies have identified multiple factors involved in MDR, and the biological processes affected by these factors vary widely, including but not limited to the efflux pump system [6], epigenetic modification [7], cell protection pathways [8, 9], oxidative stress [10], and anti-apoptotic signalling [11]. Obviously, the aetiology of MDR can be multifactorial and potentially cross-level.

One of the most common methods through which tumours acquire drug resistance involves the induction and activation of efflux transporters such as P-glycoprotein (P-gp), which affect the drug transmembrane balance at the plasma membrane [12]. Increased expression of P-gp leads to a decrease in drug accumulation in cells [13, 14]. P-gp activity can be regulated by protein phosphorylation catalysed by protein kinase C (PKC). Thus, the absorption of drugs by cancer cells is reduced [15–17].

The second mechanism that imparts drug resistance to cancer cells occurs at the intracellular level. This genetic system involves CYP3A4 [18] and glutathione-S-transferase (GST) [19], both of which are enzymes that contribute to cell detoxification and hinder the accumulation of potentially heterologous organisms in cancer cells [5]. The detoxification function of glutathione has also been shown to play an important role in the development of colon cancer resistance to 5-FU.

Magnetic resonance spectroscopy (MRS) is a noninvasive magnetic resonance imaging (MRI) technique that indirectly reflects changes in the metabolic state of living tissues and organs by measuring changes in the chemical composition of a certain area of the human body [20]. 1H-MRS is sufficiently sensitive to detect changes in key metabolites of the metabolic pathway related to the glutathione (i.e., GSH) system in the tumour [20].

Studies on gliomas (the most common type of brain tumour) have found that tumour cells increase glutamine through metabolic reprogramming to provide an abnormally depleted energy source [21, 22], suggesting that an increase in glutamine concentration is related to therapeutic resistance and proliferation of tumour [23]. MRS has been used to quantify changes in metabolites induced by metabolic reprogramming, distinguishing between proliferative gliomas and brain metastases [24, 25]. Clinical longitudinal studies in patients with glioblastomas suggested that pretreatment glutamine and glutamate levels detected by 1H-MRS in glioblastomas were correlated with tumour proliferation and poor prognosis [26].

Our study first demonstrated that 1H-MRS can detect increases in the glutamate metabolism complex (Glx1 and Glx2) in vivo in 5-FU-resistant xenograft tumours, which reflect increased glutathione biological synthesis [27]. Therefore, 1H-MRS may play an important role in the detection of molecular markers of changes in tumour resistance in vivo. In the present study, we opted to investigate the changes in GSH metabolites between 5-FU-responsive and 5-FU-resistant colon cancer tissue via in vivo 1H-MRS with 3.0 T MRI. This preliminary investigation aims to provide knowledge on the characteristic metabolites and molecular mechanisms of the drug resistance of CRC.

2. Research process

2.1 Methods

2.1.1 Cell lines and resistance index

The human colorectal adenocarcinoma cell line SW480 was obtained from the Experimental Animal Center of Sun Yat-sen University (Guangzhou, China). Its 5-FU-resistant subline, SW480/5-FU, was developed by the high-dose impact method with 5-FU (Xudong Haipu Pharmaceutical Co., Ltd., Shanghai, China) [28]. SW480/5-FU cells that were capable of stable growth in 6 μg/mL 5-FU were regarded as a 5-FU-resistant strain and named SW480/5-FU cells. Both SW480 and SW480/5-FU cells were cultured in RPMI 1640 medium (HyClone Laboratories, Logan, UT, United States) supplemented with 10% foetal bovine serum (Gibco, Invitrogen, Waltham, MA, United States) and 100 U/mL penicillin (Solarbio Life Science, Beijing, China) at 37°C in a humidified 5% CO_2 atmosphere and passaged twice a week.

MTT assays were performed to determine the relative cell viability of the parental SW480 and SW480/5-FU cells. For this assay, the cell lines were grown in RPMI 1640 medium as described above and seeded in 96-well plates at a density of 3000 cells of each cell line per well [28]. The cells were treated with 5-FU at various concentrations (0.5, 1.25, 2.5, 5, 10, 50, or 250 μg/mL) for 48 h. MTT (10 μL of 0.5 mg/mL) was added to each well, and the cells were incubated for 4 h. All liquid was removed, and 150 μL of dimethyl sulfoxide was added to each well. The absorbance at 490 nm was read using a multifunction microplate reader (Boteng Instrumentation Co., Ltd., Beijing, China).

The half-maximal inhibitory concentration (IC_{50}) of the SW480 and SW480/5-FU cells was determined using SPSS v13.0 statistical software (IBM Corp., Armonk, NY, United States). The resistance index (RI) of the SW480/5-FU cells was calculated as (SW480/5-FU IC_{50})/SW480 IC_{50} = 4.44.

2.1.2 Tumour xenograft model

All animal experiments conformed to the internationally accepted principles for the care and use of laboratory animals (Licence No. 2017-007, Ethical Committee for Animal Research of Guangzhou Medical University, China).

Five- to six-week-old BALB/c nude mice were purchased from the Guangdong Provincial Animal Experiment Center (15–17 g, females, No. 44007200046136). Ten healthy BALB/c nude mice (female, aged 5–6 weeks, 16–18 g) were randomly divided into a resistant tumour group and a responsive tumour group (5 mice in each group). Tumour xenograft models were prepared as previously described [28, 29]. Briefly, 0.2 mL of a suspension (4×10^7 cells/mL) of SW480 cells (responsive tumour group) or SW480/5-FU cells (resistant tumour group) was injected subcutaneously into the bilateral hind leg root to reduce the amount of mouse used. The animals were housed in the specific pathogen-free facility at the Animal Experimental Center of Guangzhou Medical University. Based on the ethical standard of tumor burden on mice in the "Guidelines for the welfare and use of animals in cancer research, 2010" [30], the maximal diameter of tumours on mice was limited to less than 1.5 cm.

2.1.3 In vivo MRI/1H-MRS

Immediately before the MR examination, each tumour-bearing mouse was wrapped in plastic material to provide warmth and prevent curling artifact [28]. In addition, increasing the volume of the imaged subjects can fill the coil imaging space and improve the reliability of the data collection.

MR was performed using the MAGNETOM Skyra 3 T Siemens MR Imaging System (Erlangen, Germany) equipped with an 8-channel mouse coil (Chenguang Medical Technology Co., Shanghai, China). Axial, coronal, and sagittal T2WI (TSE) images (repetition time/echo time = 4500 ms/110 ms, slice thickness = 2 mm, interval = 0, field of vision = 128 mm, NSA = 4, SENSE = 2, acquisition matrix = 128 × 128, reconstruction matrix = 512 × 512, scan time = 2 min 2 s) were acquired to determine the spectroscopic volume of interest in the cancer lesion (i.e., the hyperintense region in the images) (**Figure 1**).

1H-MRS was performed using the multivoxel three-dimensional volume acquisition editing MEGA-PRESS sequence with previously described procedures and parameters (repetition time = 1700 ms, echo time = 40 ms, slice thickness = 2 mm, interval = 0, field of vision = 60 mm, volume of interest = 30 mm, collection voxel size = 4–9 mm, acquisition number = 8, acquisition matrix = 128 × 128, scan time = 9 min 13 s) [28].

The acquired spectral data were processed using the device software (Siemens), as previously described [28], and then independently reviewed by two radiologists (Yang YM and Wu MY), who were blinded to the sample grouping [28]. Any discrepancies were resolved by discussion and consensus. The two reviewers independently determined the semiquantitative value (area under the peak) from three different voxels of the tumour while avoiding necrotic areas on T2 images; the two

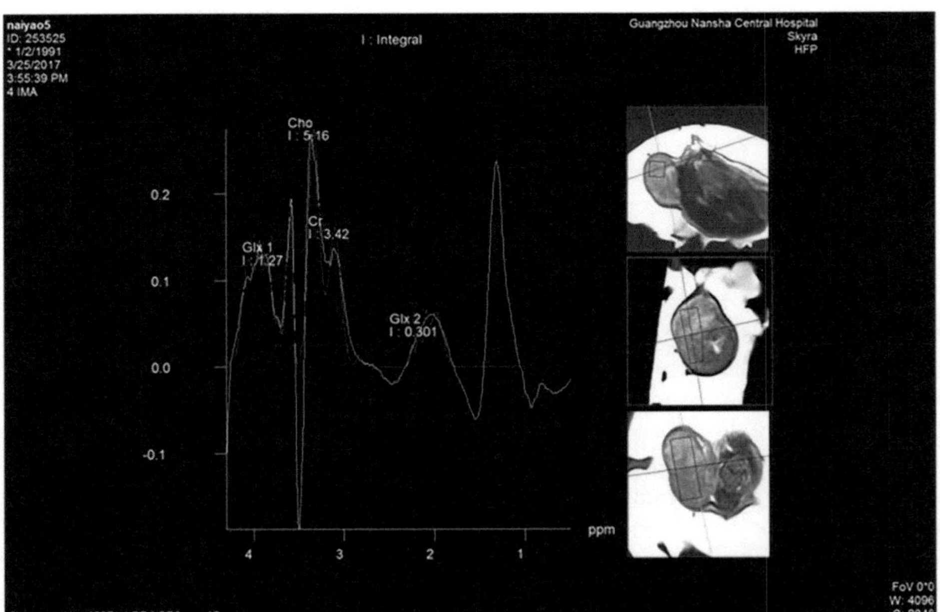

Figure 1.
Metabolic profiles of SW480/5-fluorouracil cancer tissue in vivo.

values were then averaged, and the resultant single value was used for the subsequent statistical analysis.

Choline (Cho; 3.21 ppm) and the glutamate and glutamine complex (Glx1; 2.05–2.35 ppm and Glx2; 3.75–3.8 ppm, respectively) were the target metabolites investigated in this study (**Figure 1**).

2.1.4 Cancer tissue analysis

After MRI, the tumour-bearing mice were sacrificed via the intraperitoneal injection of 10% chloral hydrate. The tumours were removed completely and prepared for histological analysis [haematoxylin-eosin (HE) staining], western blotting, and MTT assays [28].

The histopathological evaluations were performed by a pathologist with 25 years of work experience (Zhang J). Tumour necrosis was assessed using the HE-stained sections (magnification × 400). The degree of necrosis was rated on a 5-point scale: 1 (light) indicated necrosis in 1/5 of the tumour tissue, 2 (moderate) indicated necrosis in 2/5 of the tumour tissue, 3 (severe) indicated necrosis in 3/5 of the tumour tissue, 4 (very severe) indicated necrosis in 4/5 of the tumour tissue, and 5 (total) indicated necrosis throughout the entirety of the tumour tissue. The necrotic area was denoted as extremely small by a rating of 0.5 points.

Western blotting was performed to detect the expression of P-gp, multidrug resistance pump (MRP)1, PKC, γ-GCSh, γ-GCSl, glutathione synthetase (GSHS), and GST-π. Western blot testing was performed by Jie Tewei Biotechnology Co., Ltd. (Guangzhou, China) according to the instruction manual provided with the Phototope®-HRP western blot kit (Cell Signaling Technology, Danvers, MA, United States). The following antibodies were used: goat anti-mouse IgG/HRP (ABclonal, Woburn, MA, United States), MDR1 (ABclonal), MRP1 (ABclonal), PKC (ABclonal), γ-GCSh (ABclonal), γ-GCSl (ABclonal), GSHS (ABclonal), and GST-π (Cell Signaling Technology). The detected protein bands were scanned into a computer in JPG format and analysed using ImagePro-Plus 6.0 software for automatic determination of the integral optical density (IOD) of the band intensities. The IOD of the expression of each respective protein of interest was then divided by the IOD of the internal reference (GAPDH) to obtain the relative (R)IOD.

MTT assays were performed to determine the relative cell viability of cancer tissue with different concentrations of 5-FU [28]. Briefly, the tumour tissue was minced (to a size of 1–2 mm^3), suspended in 1 mL of trypsin-EDTA (Gibco), and allowed to digest for 50 min in a 37°C incubator. After the addition of 2 mL of RPMI 1640 medium (HyClone Laboratories, Logan, UT, United States) to terminate digestion, the cell suspension was separated by centrifugation (5 min at a rotation speed of 1000 r/min), resuspended in fresh RPMI 1640 medium (2–3 mL), and filtered through a 200-mesh sieve into a 25-cm^2 culture flask. The IC_{50} was measured by the MTT assay.

2.1.5 Statistical analysis

The SPSS v13.1 statistical software package was used for all the calculations. The data are summarized as the means and standard deviations. Due to the small sample size, the Mann-Whitney *U* test was selected for the comparison of metabolites and protein expression between the 5-FU-responsive group and the 5-FU-resistance group. The correlations between metabolites and P-gp, PKC, MRP1, γ-GCSl, γ-GCSh,

GSHS, and GST-π protein expression were assessed by Spearman's correlation test. A *P*-value less than 0.05 was considered to indicate statistical significance.

2.2 Results

Two tumours smaller than 1 cm were removed from each group. A total of 16 tumours were included in this study: 8 from the 5-FU-responsive (SW480) mice (maximum diameter range: 1. 21–1.48 cm) and 8 from the 5-FU-resistant (SW480/5-FU) mice (maximum diameter range: 1.15–1.46 cm).

2.2.1 Evaluation of resistance to 5-FU

2.2.1.1 SW480/5-FU cells exhibit higher survivability in cancer tissue in vivo than the parental SW480 cells

The viability of both the parental SW480 cells and SW480/5-FU cells decreased with increases in the concentrations of 5-FU (**Figure 2**, MTT). The SW480/5-FU tumours exhibited a significantly higher survival rate than the SW480 tumours ($P < 0.05$) when the 5-FU concentration was higher than 2.5 μg/mL. The RI of SW480/5-FU cells was calculated as follows: (SW480/5-FU IC_{50})/SW480 IC_{50} = 42.914 μg/mL/9.516 μg/mL = 4.508.

2.2.1.2 The SW480/5-FU xenograft tumours showed significantly higher expression of resistance-related proteins

The SW480/5-FU xenograft tumours showed higher expression of P-gp, MRP1, and PKC than the SW480 xenograft tumours (**Figures 3** and **4**). A statistical comparison of the RIOD values obtained for the expression of these proteins between the two groups revealed that the difference was significant; the Mann-Whitney *U* test *Z* and *P* values for P-gp, MRP1, and KPC were 2.611 and 0.003, 2.785 and 0.005, and 2.668 and 0.008, respectively.

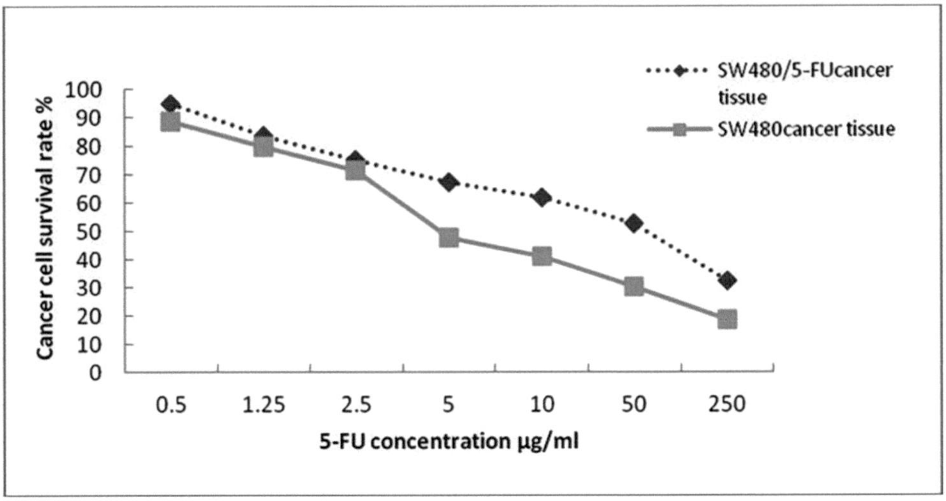

Figure 2.
Drug resistance curves of SW480/5-fluorouracil and SW480 xenograft tumours.

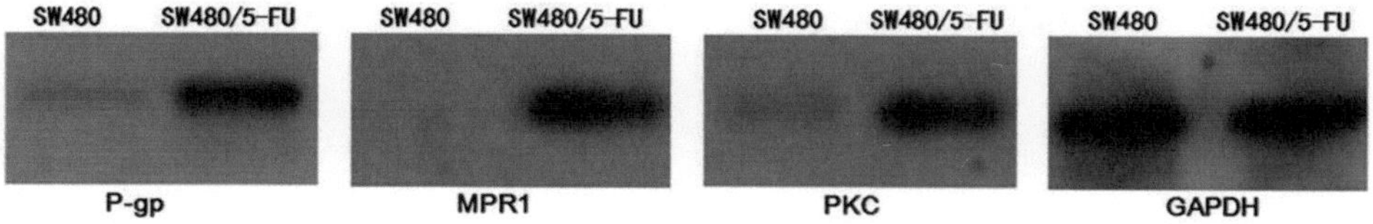

Figure 3.
Expression of P-glycoprotein, multidrug resistance pump 1, and protein kinase C in SW480/5-fluorouracil xenograft tumours and SW480 xenograft tumours.

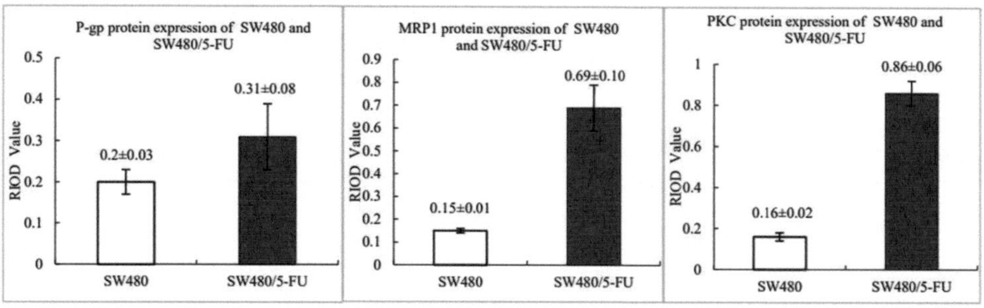

Figure 4.
Relative integral optical density values for the expression levels of P-glycoprotein, multidrug resistance pump 1, and protein kinase C in SW480/5-fluorouracil xenograft tumours and SW480 xenograft tumours.

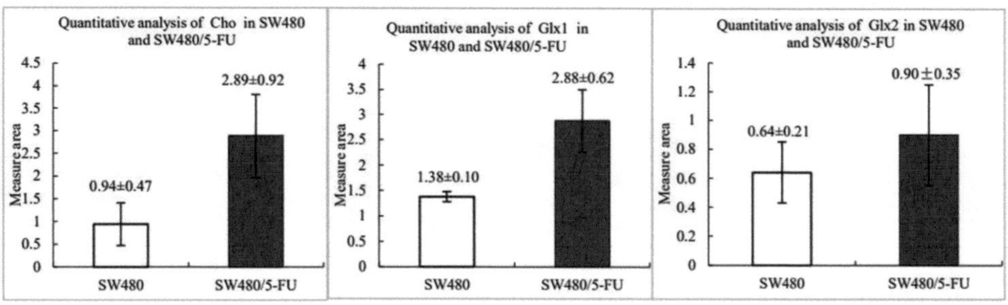

Figure 5.
Peak areas of choline, glutamate, and glutamine complex in the SW480/5-fluorouracil xenograft tumours and SW480 xenograft tumours.

2.2.2 1H-MRS analysis

The SW480 (5-FU responsive) and SW480/5-FU (5-FU resistant) tumour tissues were assessed by 1H-MRS for the *in vivo* detection of Cho, Glx1, and Glx2 peaks. The areas under the peak values for each of these metabolites are summarized in **Figure 5**. All three metabolites were found at significantly higher levels in the 5-FU-resistant tumours, as determined by the Mann-Whitney *U* test.

2.2.3 Cancer tissue analysis

2.2.3.1 Tumour necrosis

No significant difference in the degree of necrosis was observed between the HE-stained tumour tissues of the SW480 (5-FU responsive) and SW480/5-FU

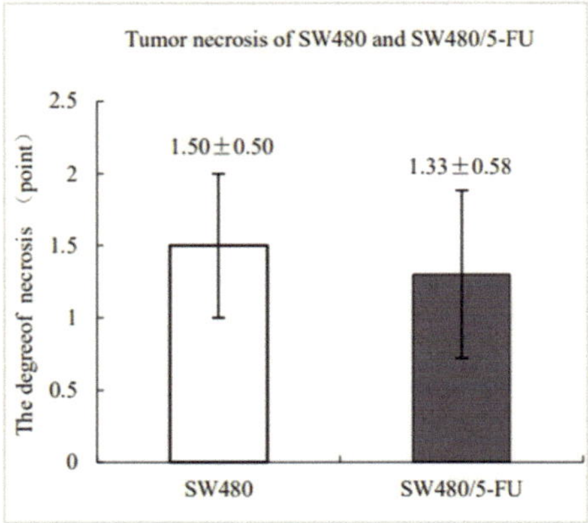

Figure 6.
Degree of necrosis in the SW480/5-fluorouracil xenograft tumours and SW480 xenograft tumours.

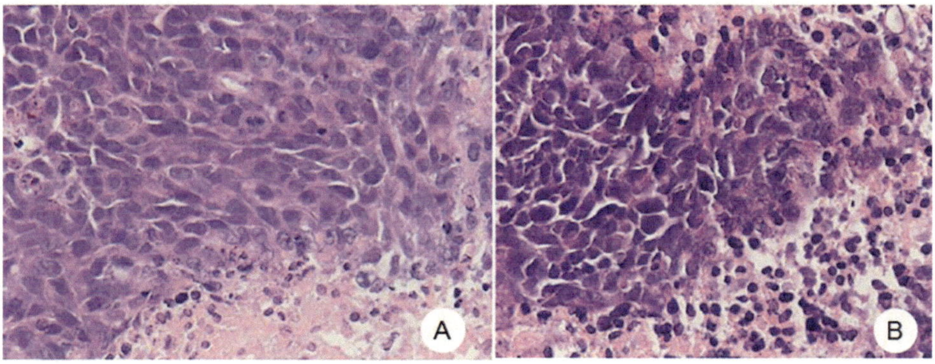

Figure 7.
Haematoxylin-eosin staining analysis of tumour tissues. Haematoxylin-eosin staining analysis of tumour tissues (magnification: 400×).

(5-FU resistant) xenografts (**Figure 6**; T tests, t = 1.76, P = 0.109). However, differences in other histological features were observed. The SW480/5-FU (5-FU resistant) tumour tissues showed larger cell nuclei, a closer cell arrangement, and a greater cell density (**Figure** 7).

2.2.3.2 Expression of γ-GCSh, γ-GCSl, GSHS, and GST-π proteins in tumour tissues

The SW480/5-FU (5-FU resistant) tumour tissues showed higher expression of glutamate-metabolizing enzyme proteins than the SW480 (5-FU responsive) tumour tissues (**Figures 8** and **9**). A statistical comparison of the RIOD values for the expression levels of these proteins between the two groups revealed that the difference was significant; specifically, the Mann-Whitney U test Z and P values for γ-GCSh, γ-GCSl, GSHS, and GST-π were 2.643 and 0.008, 2.712 and 0.007, 2.635 and 0.008, and 2.627 and 0.008, respectively.

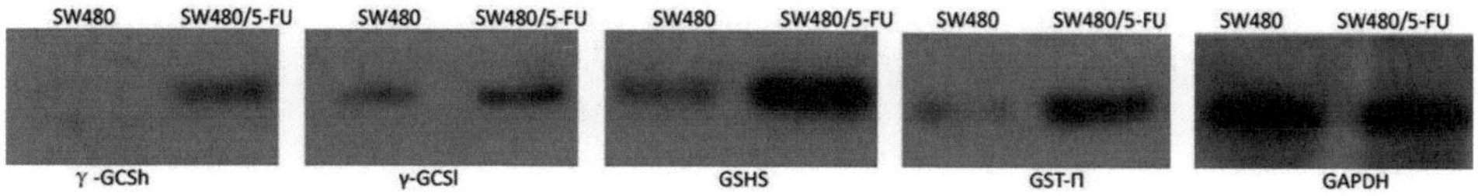

Figure 8.
Expression of γ-GCSh, γ-GCSl, glutathione synthetase, and glutathione-π in SW480/5-fluorouracil xenograft tumours and SW480 xenograft tumours.

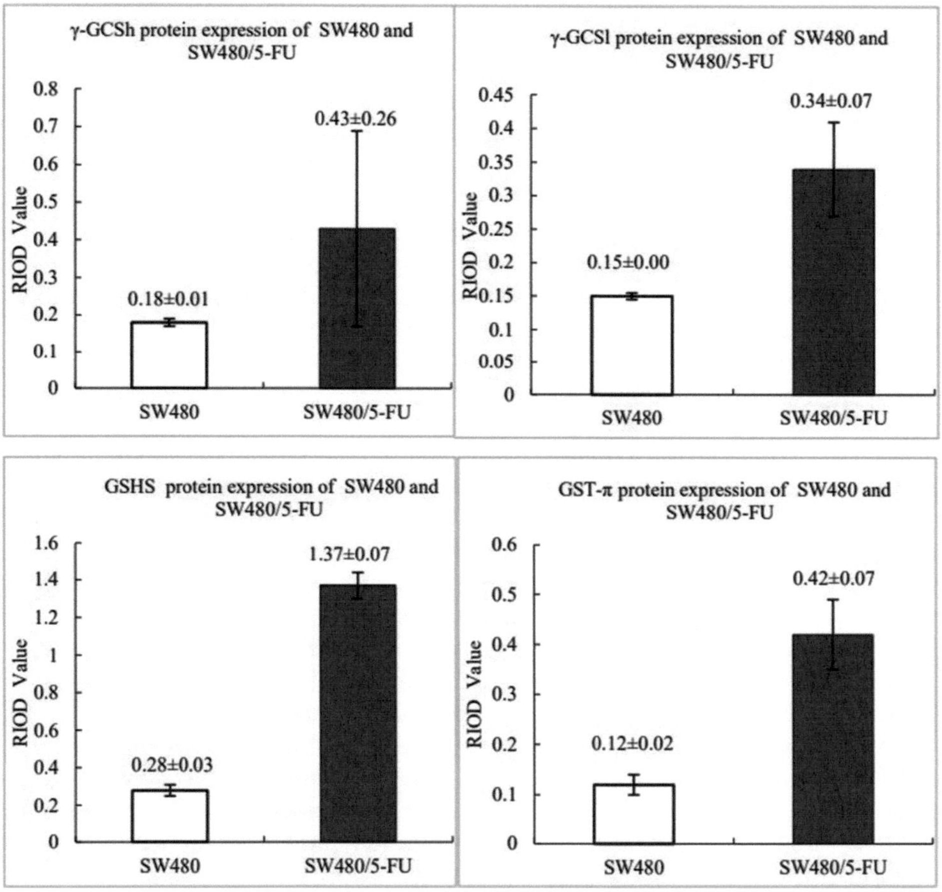

Figure 9.
Relative integral optical density values for the expression levels of γ-GCSh, γ-GCSl, glutathione synthetase, and glutathione-π in SW480/5-fluorouracil xenograft tumours and SW480 xenograft tumours.

2.2.4 Correlation between metabolites detected by 1H-MRS and protein expression in tumour cells

The Cho peak area was positively correlated with the expression of P-gp (r = 0.636, P = 0.048), MRP1 (r = 0.821, P = 0.004), γ-GCSh (r = 0.841, P = 0.002), and γ-GCSl (r = 0.799, P = 0.006). The Glx1 peak area was positively correlated with the expression of MRP1 (r = 0.880, P = 0.021) and GST-π (r = 0.888, P = 0.018), and the Glx2 peak area exhibited positive correlations with the expression of

MRP1 ($r = 0.847$, $P = 0.002$), γ-GCSh ($r = 0.644$, $P = 0.044$), γ-GCShl ($r = 0.780$, $P = 0.008$), and GSHS ($r = 0.661$, $P = 0.038$).

2.3 Discussion

In this study, the high-dose shock method was used to obtain 5-FU-resistant cells from 5-FU-responsive cells, i.e., SW480/5-FU cells from parental SW480 cells. The RI of the SW480/5-FU cells *in vitro* was very close to that of cancer tissue created with these cells in a xenograft mouse model. The SW480/5-FU tumour tissues showed significantly increased expression of P-gp, MRP1, and PKC, which indicated the reliable features of these cells for the *in vivo* study of 5-FU resistance. At the same time, it was also observed that there was no difference in the necrotic range between 5-FU-resistant and 5-FU-responsive colon cancer tissues before being attacked by 50-FU. However, 5-FU-resistant colon cancer tissues had larger nuclei and higher cell density, indicating a significant difference in their proliferative ability. It is speculated that the related metabolites supporting the stronger proliferative ability of 5-FU-resistant colon cancer are higher.

During the development of drug resistance, a harsh microenvironment containing chemotherapeutic drugs will induce tumour cells to undergo metabolic reorganization at the genetic level (i.e., gene mutations in the cell cycle pathway) [31–33] up to the protein level (i.e., mutation of metabolic enzymes) [34]. This reorganization results in changes in the metabolite composition of the tumor and surrounding tissues [33, 35]. Eventually, the microenvironment itself may become beneficial to tumour survival. The related changes in the levels of certain metabolites will then differentiate chemotherapy-responsive tumours from chemotherapy-resistant tumours. Such metabolites represent the last step in the biological process of the tumour towards immortality, but the clinical measurement of such metabolites can provide insight into the case and its prognosis and/or management.

Compounds in human tissues can produce quantifiable chemical shifts under specific conditions. The peak value generated by these shifts can be determined by 1H-MRS, and the area or peak height of compound resonance peaks can be calculated to quantify the content of compounds in a tissue [36–39]. Thus, 1H-MRS can detect metabolite changes before and after the development of multidrug resistance in tumour tissues in vivo and is particularly useful for screening metabolites with detoxification functions that can improve the tumour microenvironment. We based our study on this speculation that 1H-MRS has potential value for detecting tumour resistance in vivo.

GSH is a small-molecule peptide composed of three amino acids (tripeptide thiol). Its main function is to detoxify and remove xenobiotics and other endogenous compounds from the cell [27]. As such, its antioxidant function is closely related to tumour MDR, which is an important feature of the drug resistance of malignant tumours [40]. A large amount of reactive oxygen species (ROS) is produced during tumour metabolism. High levels of ROS are cytotoxic and can cause apoptosis. Due to the growth characteristics of tumour cells, these cells exist in a state of low oxygen stress for a long time, which should sensitize the cells to death under the action of ROS [21, 40, 41]. Indeed, this feature serves as the basis of many chemotherapeutic drugs used in clinical practice (i.e., the achievement of an antitumour effect by generating a large amount of ROS). However, the main role of GSH is to reduce potentially toxic oxidants, such as ROS, to produce oxidized GSH in the form of glutathione disulfide (GSSG) [27] and thereby directly remove ROS from tumour cells, which unfortunately leads to drug resistance [21, 41].

In addition, anticancer drugs in tumour tissues can interact with GSH via GST and then be exported from the cells through MRP [40, 42]. MRP is a relatively large transmembrane protein and is an ATP-driven outlet pump that excludes GSSG and various glutathione-S conjugates [40, 42, 43]. Therefore, GSH improves the unfavourable microenvironment for tumour cells and increases the chances of tumour survival.

Glutamine is converted into glutamic acid under the action of glutaminase, and glutamic acid then combines with glycine to produce glutamylcysteine. This product is further combined with cysteine to form GSH by a reaction catalysed by GSHS [27]. Therefore, two key enzyme-catalysed reactions occur upstream of GSH biosynthesis.

γ-GCS is the key enzyme of the first step of GSH biosynthesis and is composed of a γ-GCSh heavy chain subunit (73 kDa) and a γ-GCSl light chain subunit (27.7 kDa) [27, 44]. γ-GCSh harbours all functions of the complete catalytic enzyme and can independently catalyse GSH synthesis without the γ-GCSl subunit, which is regulated by GSH feedback [45]. In contrast, the γ-GCSl subunit harbours no enzymatic activity but can combine with the γ-GCSh subunit through noncovalent bonds to form a holoenzyme, which changes the spatial structure of γ-GCSh and enhances its catalytic activity [46]. Compared with the results obtained with γ-GCSh alone, the catalytic activity of γ-GCSh combined with γ-GCSl is higher and is less suppressed by GSH feedback [47].

GSHS is the second key enzyme in GSH biosynthesis [27]. GSHS, which is composed of two subunits and has the same molecular weight as γ-glutamylcysteine synthetase, is not subject to feedback regulation by GSH [27]. It has been reported that GSHS is less important in GSH biosynthesis than γ-GCS [47]. However, another study demonstrated that GSHS plays a decisive role in GSH synthesis under certain tissue hypoxia conditions [48]. Hamdoum et al. [49] reported that the synthesis of GSH is reduced in response to treatment with GSHS inhibitors, which benefits leukaemia patients by increasing their sensitivity to chemotherapy drugs.

GST represents a group of isozymes that exists in a broad array of organisms, is encoded by multiple genes, and has myriad physiological functions [40]. Some studies have shown that the abnormal expression of GST isoenzymes is related to the metabolism of anticancer drugs that results in tumour drug resistance [50–53]. The GST gene family is a huge supergene family. In terms of phenotype, each type of isozyme includes many subtypes, and there are five subtypes [54]. Some studies have found that GST-π exhibits the closest relationship with tumour MDR [54]. GST-π is a phase II metabolic enzyme that is expressed at high levels in most tumour cells [55–58]. GST-π can catalyse the binding of harmful biological ions from internal and external sources to GSH, which protects cells from damage. The GSH-chemotherapeutic drug conjugate is actively pumped out of cells through MRP1, which reduces the accumulation of chemotherapeutic drugs in cells [40, 43]. GST-π can also be combined with some anticancer drugs to form a complex with higher water solubility and easier excretion. The complex is excreted through the kidneys, which reduces the cytotoxicity of antitumour drugs but can also cause MDR [21]. In addition, the combination of GST-π and c-Jun N-terminal kinase impedes tumour cell apoptosis by blocking the mitogen-activated protein kinase pathway, which ultimately leads to tumour drug resistance [21].

GSH has three spin systems generated from three amino acid residues, i.e., γ-glutamyl, cysteine, and glycine. These systems are tightly coupled second-order γ-glutamyl αCH, βCH2 and γCH2, cysteine αCH and βCH2, and glycine αCH2 [59, 60]. The GSH spectrum consists of a series of resonances from the peptide components, which are more or less transferred from the separated peptide resonances.

In the central nervous system, all signals from GSH overlap with resonance from other neurochemicals. These chemicals include N-acetylaspartate (at 2.02 ppm and 2.45 ppm), polyglutamate recombination (centred at 2.05 ppm and 2.35 ppm), creatine plus creatine phosphate (at 3.03 ppm and 3.96 ppm), and amino acids such as glutamic acid, glutamine, and aspartic acid (at 3.75–3.8 ppm) [27].

In the current study, the 1H-MRS spectrum collected by clinical medical MR mainly reflects GSH and upstream metabolites, i.e., glutamine and the glutamate complex (Glx) at 2.1–2.5 ppm (CH2-CH2β-γ peak) and 3.7–3.9 ppm (α peak of amino acid CH). These complexes include the glutamate complex centred at 2.05 ppm and 2.35 ppm (Glx1) and amino acids such as glutamic acid, glutamine, and aspartic acid at 3.75–3.8 ppm (Glx2). The GLX peak detected in vivo using 1H-MRS indirectly reflects the metabolic changes of GSH [27].

This study found that γ-GCSh, γ-GCSl, GSHS, and GST were significantly increased in SW480/5-FU tumour tissues compared with SW480 tumour tissues, which indicated that the functions of GSH synthesis, detoxification, and removal of xenobiotics and other endogenous compounds increased and resulted in tumour tissue resistance to 5-FU. In addition, the peak areas of Glx1 and Glx2 detected by 1H-MRS in vivo in the SW480/5-FU tumour tissues were significantly higher than those found in the SW480 tumour tissues. The area of Glx1 was highly positively correlated with the expression of MRP1 and GST-π, and the area of Glx2 was highly positively correlated with the expression of MRP1, γ-GCSh, γ-GCShl, and GSHS. Therefore, the biological processes of GSH synthesis and detoxification can be reproduced in vivo, which suggests the formation of tumour resistance.

This study also showed that the cell nuclei of SW480/5-FU tumour cells were larger than those of SW480 tumour cells (by HE histology); in addition, the former cells were arranged more closely and exhibited a higher cell density. These findings indicate that drug-resistant tumour cells proliferate more actively. The area of the Cho peak detected with 1H-MRS in vivo was also significantly higher with SW480/5-FU tumour cells and was positively correlated with the expression of tumour P-gp, MRP1, γ-GCSh, and γ-GCSl. The level of Cho is closely related to Cho and phospholipid metabolic activities, and the phospholipid bilayer is the basis of the cell membrane. Thus, the Cho levels can indirectly reflect the activity of cell membrane metabolism [61, 62]. We hypothesize that Cho may be able to promote or synergize with GSH synthetic biological processes.

Our study has inherent limitations that must be considered when interpreting our findings. First, only eight samples per group were included in this study. Further study with a larger sample size is needed to determine the stability and repeatability of the observed indicators. Second, the collection of 1H-MRS data for tumours in xenograft models with clinical medical MRI systems may lead to a low signal-to-noise ratio and result in bias. In addition, MRS remains a limited research tool. The relatively long acquisition time is currently difficult to standardize and complicates the accurate quantification of the metabolite tissue concentration [27]. This study constitutes preliminary exploratory research using a 3 T MRI system equipped with an 8-channel mouse coil, and we found a preliminary experimental result. Therefore, an ultra-high field small animal MRI system with higher than 7 T is needed to verify the repeatability and reliability of 1H-MRS for metabolite data acquisition. Finally, we only studied 5-FU-resistant colon cancer, but other clinical chemotherapeutic drugs for colon cancer were not included. The addition of an experimental exploration of resistance to other clinical chemotherapeutic drugs for colon cancer, such as FOLFOX, 5-FU/LV, and other treatment regimens at the preclinical stage, is needed.

DOI: http://dx.doi.org/10.5772/intechopen.1004157

3. Conclusion

1H-MRS can detect increases in Glx1 and Glx2 metabolites, reflecting an increase in the GSH biological synthesis process, which is a cause of drug resistance in tumours. Active membrane metabolism of tumours, tumour acidification, and GSH synthesis biological processes have a promoting or synergistic effect, and the possible mechanisms and connections need to be explored further. Therefore, 1H-MRS is expected to provide biomarkers for the evaluation of colon cancer drug resistance by detecting changes in tumour metabolites *in vivo*.

Acknowledgements

This work was supported by the Natural Science Foundation of Guangdong [No. 2015A030313732] and the Guangzhou Science and Technology Plan Project (No. 201907010020).

The authors would like to express their gratitude to Wei-Ling Huang and Qi-Feng Pan for the technical assistance provided with the MRI.

Conflict of interest

The authors declare no conflict of interest.

Author details

Qi Xie[1*], Yi-Ming Yang[2], Min-Yi Wu[3], Xi-Yan Shao[4], Gui-Qin Wang[5] and Jing Zhang[6]

1 Medical Imaging Department in Nansha, Guangzhou First People's Hospital, School of Medicine, South China University of Technology, Guangzhou, China

2 Department of Radiology, Guangdong Provincial Hospital of Traditional Chinese Medicine, Guangzhou University of Traditional Chinese Medicine, Guangzhou, China

3 Department of Radiology, Panyu Central Hospital of Guangzhou, Guangzhou, China

4 Medical Imaging Department, The Second Affiliated Hospital, School of Medicine, The Chinese University of Hong Kong (Shenzhen), Shenzhen, China

5 Medical Record Department in Nansha, Guangzhou First People's Hospital, School of Medicine, South China University of Technology, Guangzhou, China

6 Department of Pathology, Cancer Center, Sun Yat-sen University, Guangzhou, China

*Address all correspondence to: eyqixie@scut.edu.cn

References

[1] Douillard JY, Cunningham D, Roth AD, Navarro M, James RD, Karasek P, et al. Irinotecan combined with fluorouracil compared with fluorouracil alone as first-line treatment for metastatic colorectal cancer: A multicentre randomised trial. Lancet. 2000;**355**:1041-1047. DOI: 10.1016/s0140-6736 (00)02034-1

[2] Soerjomataram I, Lortet-Tieulent J, Parkin DM, Ferlay J, Mathers C, Forman D, et al. Global burden of cancer in 2008: A systematic analysis of disability-adjusted life-years in 12 world regions. Lancet. 2012;**380**:1840-1850. DOI: 10.1016/S0140-6736(12)60919-2

[3] Brenner H, Kloor M, Pox CP. Colorectal cancer. Lancet. 2014;**26: 383**(9927):1490-1502. DOI: 10.1016/S0140-6736(13)61649-9

[4] Li Y, Gong P, Hou JX, Huang W, Ma XP, Wang YL, et al. miR-34a regulates multidrug resistance via positively modulating OAZ2 signaling in colon cancer cells. Journal of Immunology Research. 2018;**2018**:7498514. DOI: 10.1155/2018/7498514

[5] Li T, Jia YM, Lei KJ. Summary of drug sensitivity assay of tumor cells in vitro. Journal of Modern Oncology. 2016;**24**:828-830. DOI: 10.3969/j.issn.1672-4992.2016.05.043

[6] Liu YR, Liang L, Zhao JM, Zhang Y, Zhang M, Zhong WL, et al. Twist1 confers multidrug resistance in colon cancer through upregulation of ATP-binding cassette transporters. Oncotarget. 2017;**8**:52901-52912. DOI: 10.18632/oncotarget.17548

[7] Calcagno AM, Fostel JM, To KK, Salcido CD, Martin SE, Chewning KJ, et al. Single-step doxorubicin-selected cancer cells overexpress the ABCG2 drug transporter through epigenetic changes. British Journal of Cancer. 2008;**98**:1515-1524. DOI: 10.1038/sj.bjc.6604334

[8] Lubelska K, Wiktorska K, Mielczarek L, Milczarek M, Zbroińska-Bregisz I, Chilmonczyk Z. Sulforaphane regulates NFE2L2/Nrf2-dependent xenobiotic metabolism phase II and phase III enzymes differently in human colorectal cancer and untransformed epithelial colon cells. Nutrition and Cancer. 2016;**68**:1338-1348. DOI: 10.1080/01635581.2016.1224369

[9] Ebert B, Kisiela M, Wsól V, Maser E. Proteasome inhibitors MG-132 and bortezomib induce AKR1C1, AKR1C3, AKR1B1, and AKR1B10 in human colon cancer cell lines SW-480 and HT-29. Chemico-Biological Interactions. 2011;**191**:239-249. DOI: 10.1016/j.cbi.2010.12.026

[10] Šemeláková M, Jendželovský R, Fedoročko P. Drug membrane transporters and CYP3A4 are affected by hypericin, hyperforin or aristoforin in colon adenocarcinoma cells. Biomedicine & Pharmacotherapy. 2016;**81**:38-47. DOI: 10.1016/j.biopha.2016.03.045

[11] Xiang Z, Kang QJ, Xiang X. Gene and protein expression in the oxaliplatin-resistant HT29/L-OHP human colon cancer cell line. Genetics and Molecular Research. 2015;**14**:11013-11022. DOI: 10.4238/2015.September.21.14

[12] El-Readi MZ, Eid S, Abdelghany AA, Al-Amoudi HS, Efferth T, Wink M. Resveratrol mediated cancer cell apoptosis, and modulation of multidrug resistance proteins and metabolic

enzymes. Phytomedicine. 2019;**55**:269-281. DOI: 10.1016/j.phymed.2018.06.046

[13] Meijerman I, Beijnen JH, Schellens JH. Combined action and regulation of phase II enzymes and multidrug resistance proteins in multidrug resistance in cancer. Cancer Treatment Reviews. 2008;**34**:505-520. DOI: 10.1016/j.ctrv.2008.03.002

[14] Gillet JP, Gottesman MM. Mechanisms of multidrug resistance in cancer. Methods in Molecular Biology. 2010;**596**:47-76. DOI: 10.1007/978-1-60761-416-6_4

[15] Hu YP, Robert J. Inhibition of protein kinase C in multidrug-resistant cells by modulators of multidrug resistance. Journal of Cancer Research and Clinical Oncology. 1997;**123**:201-210. DOI: 10.1007/BF01240316

[16] Kim CW, Asai D, Kang JH, Kishimura A, Mori T, Katayama Y. Reversal of efflux of an anticancer drug in human drug-resistant breast cancer cells by inhibition of protein kinase Cα (PKCα) activity. Tumour Biology. 2016;**37**:1901-1908. DOI: 10.1007/s13277-015-3963-4

[17] Fang Z, Xu A, Wu L, Hei TK, Hong M. The role of protein kinase C alpha translocation in radiation-induced bystander effect. Scientific Reports. 2016;**6**:25817. DOI: 10.1038/srep25817

[18] Gupta A, Mugundu GM, Desai PB, Thummel KE, Unadkat JD. Intestinal human colon adenocarcinoma cell line LS180 is an excellent model to study pregnane X receptor, but not constitutive androstane receptor, mediated CYP3A4 and multidrug resistance transporter 1 induction: Studies with anti-human immunodeficiency virus protease inhibitors. Drug Metabolism and Disposition. 2008;**36**:1172-1180. DOI: 10.1124/dmd.107.018689

[19] Kano T, Sakai M, Muramatsu M. Structure and expression of a human class pi glutathione S-transferase messenger RNA. Cancer Research. 1987;**47**:5626-5630

[20] Rae CD, Williams SR. Glutathione in the human brain: Review of its roles and measurement by magnetic resonance spectroscopy. Analytical Biochemistry. 2017;**529**:127-143. DOI: 10.1016/j.ab.2016.12.022

[21] Hensley CT, Wasti AT, DeBerardinis RJ. Glutamine and cancer: Cell biology, physiology, and clinical opportunities. The Journal of Clinical Investigation. 2013;**123**:3678-3684. DOI: 10.1172/JCI69600

[22] Márquez J, Alonso FJ, Matés JM, Segura JA, Martín-Rufián M, Campos-Sandoval JA. Glutamine addiction in gliomas. Neurochemical Research. 2017;**42**:1735-1746. DOI: 10.1007/s11064-017-2212-1

[23] Ekici S, Nye JA, Neill SG, Allen JW, Shu HK, Fleischer CC. Glutamine imaging: A new avenue for glioma management. American Journal of Neuroradiology. 2022;**43**:11-18. DOI: 10.3174/ajnr.A7333

[24] Cordova JS, Shu HK, Liang Z, Gurbani SS, Cooper LA, Holder CA, et al. Whole-brain spectroscopic MRI biomarkers identify infiltrating margins in glioblastoma patients. Neuro-Oncology. 2016;**18**:1180-1189. DOI: 10.1093/neuonc/now036

[25] Ohba S, Murayama K, Abe M, Hasegawa M, Hirose Y. Magnetic resonance imaging and proton magnetic resonance spectroscopy for differentiating between enhanced gliomas and malignant lymphomas. World Neurosurgery. 2019;**127**:e779-e787. DOI: 10.1016/j.wneu.2019.03.261

[26] Heintz A, Chombar J, Boussida S, Saidak Z, Lefranc M, Deleval N, et al. P14.92 study of glutaminergic and glutamatergic metabolism in 1H-MRS monovoxel in the most aggressive part of 62 glioblastoma before and after 18 months treatment. Neuro-Oncology. 2019;**21**(Suppl 3):iii89. DOI: 10.1093/neuonc/noz126.327

[27] Xie Q, Chen HX, Du L, Liao YH, Tan ZL, Yang YM, et al. Detection of the drug resistance of human colon cancer in mice with Proton Magnetic Resonance Spectroscopy. China Journal of Magnetic Resonance Imaging. 2019;**10**:435-439. DOI: 10.12015/issn.1674-8034.2019.06

[28] Yang YM. In vivo detection of the drug resistance of human colon cancer in mice with intravoxel incoherent motion diffusion imaging and proton magnetic resonance spectrum [thesis]. Guangzhou: Guangzhou Medical University; 2017

[29] Xie Q, Wu MY, Zhang DX, Yang YM, Wang BS, Zhang J, et al. Synergistic anticancer effect of exogenous wild-type p53 gene combined with 5-FU in human colon cancer resistant to 5-FU in vivo. World Journal of Gastroenterology. 2016;**22**:7342-7352. DOI: 10.3748/wjg.v22.i32.7342

[30] Workman P, AboagyeE O, Balkwill F, Balmain A, Bruder G, Chaplin DJ, et al. Committee of the National Cancer Research Institute: Guidelines for the welfare and use of animals in cancer research. British Journal of Cancer. 2010;**102**:1555-1577. DOI: 10.1038/sj.bjc.6605642

[31] Otto AM. Warburg effect(s)-a biographical sketch of Otto Warburg and his impacts on tumour metabolism. Cancer & Metabolism. 2016;**4**:5. DOI: 10.1186/s40170-016-0145-9

[32] Wolpaw AJ, Dang CV. MYC-induced metabolic stress and tumorigenesis. Biochimica Et Biophysica Acta. Reviews on Cancer. 2018;**1870**:43-50. DOI: 10.1016/j.bbcan.2018.05.003

[33] Dowell AC, Cobby E, Wen K, Devall AJ, During V, Anderson J, et al. Interleukin-17-positive mast cells influence outcomes from BCG for patients with CIS: Data from a comprehensive characterisation of the immune microenvironment of urothelial bladder cancer. PLoS One. 2017;**12**:e0184841. DOI: 10.1371/journal.pone.0184841

[34] Srinivasan R, Ricketts CJ, Sourbier C, Linehan WM. New strategies in renal cell carcinoma: Targeting the genetic and metabolic basis of disease. Clinical Cancer Research. 2015;**21**:10-17. DOI: 10.1158/1078-0432.CCR-13-2993

[35] Yang G, Shen W, Zhang Y, Liu M, Zhang L, Liu Q, et al. Accumulation of myeloid-derived suppressor cells (MDSCs) induced by low levels of IL-6 correlates with poor prognosis in bladder cancer. Oncotarget. 2017;**8**:38378-38388. DOI: 10.18632/oncotarget.16386

[36] Fardanesh R, Marino MA, Avendano D, Leithner D, Pinker K, Thakur SB. Proton MR spectroscopy in the breast: Technical innovations and clinical applications. Journal of Magnetic Resonance Imaging. 2019;**50**:1033-1046. DOI: 10.1002/jmri.26700

[37] Bulik M, Jancalek R, Vanicek J, Skoch A, Mechl M. Potential of MR spectroscopy for assessment of glioma grading. Clinical Neurology and Neurosurgery. 2013;**115**:146-153. DOI: 10.1016/j.clineuro.2012.11.002

[38] Bolan PJ. Magnetic resonance spectroscopy of the breast: Current status. Magnetic Resonance Imaging

Clinics of North America. 2013;**21**:625-639. DOI: 10.1016/j.mric.2013.04.008

[39] Kobus T, van der Laak JA, Maas MC, Hambrock T, Bruggink CC, Hulsbergen-van de Kaa CA, et al. Contribution of histopathologic tissue composition to quantitative MR spectroscopy and diffusion-weighted imaging of the prostate. Radiology. 2016;**278**:801-811. DOI: 10.1148/radiol.2015142889

[40] Singh S, Khan AR, Gupta AK. Role of glutathione in cancer pathophysiology and therapeutic interventions. Journal of Experimental Therapeutics & Oncology. 2012;**9**:303-316

[41] Lukey MJ, Katt WP, Cerione RA. Targeting amino acid metabolism for cancer therapy. Drug Discovery Today. 2017;**22**:796-804. DOI: 10.1016/j.drudis.2016.12.003

[42] Dringen R, Brandmann M, Hohnholt MC, Blumrich EM. Glutathione-dependent detoxification processes in astrocytes. Neurochemical Research. 2015;**40**:2570-2582. DOI: 10.1007/s11064-014-1481-1

[43] Minich T, Riemer J, Schulz JB, Wielinga P, Wijnholds J, Dringen R. The multidrug resistance protein 1 (Mrp1), but not Mrp5, mediates export of glutathione and glutathione disulfide from brain astrocytes. Journal of Neurochemistry. 2006;**97**:373-384. DOI: 10.1111/j.1471-4159.2006.03737.x

[44] Sun X, Shih AY, Johannssen HC, Erb H, Li P, Murphy TH. Two-photon imaging of glutathione levels in intact brain indicates enhanced redox buffering in developing neurons and cells at the cerebrospinal fluid and blood-brain interface. The Journal of Biological Chemistry. 2006;**281**:17420-17431. DOI: 10.1074/jbc.M601567200

[45] Dahl EL, Mulcahy RT. Cell-type specific differences in glutamate cysteine ligase transcriptional regulation demonstrate independent subunit control. Toxicological Sciences. 2001;**61**:265-272. DOI: 10.1093/toxsci/61.2.265

[46] Syu JP, Chi JT, Kung HN. Nrf2 is the key to chemotherapy resistance in MCF7 breast cancer cells under hypoxia. Oncotarget. 2016;**7**:14659-14672. DOI: 10.18632/oncotarget.7406

[47] Meister A. Glutathione synthesis. Enzymes. 1974;**10**:671-697. DOI: 10.1016/S1874-6047(08)60154-7

[48] Lu SC. Regulation of glutathione synthesis. Molecular Aspects of Medicine. 2009;**30**:42-59. DOI: 10.1016/j.mam.2008.05.005

[49] Hamdoun S, Jung P, Efferth T. Drug repurposing of the anthelmintic niclosamide to treat multidrug-resistant Leukemia. Frontiers in Pharmacology. 2017;**8**:110. DOI: 10.3389/fphar.2017.00110

[50] Dong SC, Sha HH, Xu XY, Hu TM, Lou R, Li H, et al. Glutathione S-transferase π: A potential role in antitumor therapy. Drug Design, Development and Therapy. 2018;**12**:3535-3547. DOI: 10.2147/DDDT.S169833

[51] van Gisbergen MW, Cebula M, Zhang J, Ottosson-Wadlund A, Dubois L, Lambin P, et al. Chemical reactivity window determines prodrug efficiency toward glutathione transferase overexpressing cancer cells. Molecular Pharmaceutics. 2016;**13**:2010-2025. DOI: 10.1021/acs.molpharmaceut.6b00140

[52] Liu H, Yang Z, Zang L, Wang G, Zhou S, Jin G, et al. Downregulation of glutathione S-transferase A1 suppressed

tumor growth and induced cell apoptosis in A549 cell line. Oncology Letters. 2018;**16**:467-474. DOI: 10.3892/ol.2018.8608

[53] Kulaksiz-Erkmen G, Dalmizrak O, Dincsoy-Tuna G, Dogan A, Ogus IH, Ozer N. Amitriptyline may have a supportive role in cancer treatment by inhibiting glutathione S-transferase pi (GST-π) and alpha (GST-α). Journal of Enzyme Inhibition and Medicinal Chemistry. 2013;**28**:131-136. DOI: 10.3109/14756366.2011.639017

[54] Nebert DW, Vasiliou V. Analysis of the glutathione S-transferase (GST) gene family. Human Genomics. 2004;**1**:460-464. DOI: 10.1186/1479-7364-1-6-460

[55] Karpusas M, Axarli I, Chiniadis L, Papakyriakou A, Bethanis K, Scopelitou K, et al. The interaction of the chemotherapeutic drug chlorambucil with human glutathione transferase A1-1: Kinetic and structural analysis. PLoS One. 2013;**8**:e56337. DOI: 10.1371/journal.pone.0056337

[56] Ye ZW, Zhang J, Ancrum T, Manevich Y, Townsend DM, Tew KD. Glutathione S-transferase P-mediated protein S-glutathionylation of resident endoplasmic reticulum proteins influences sensitivity to drug-induced unfolded protein response. Antioxidants & Redox Signaling. 2017;**26**:247-261. DOI: 10.1089/ars.2015.6486

[57] Pljesa-Ercegovac M, Savic-Radojevic A, Matic M, Coric V, Djukic T, Radic T, et al. Glutathione transferases: Potential targets to overcome chemoresistance in solid tumors. International Journal of Molecular Sciences. 2018;**19**:3785. DOI: 10.3390/ijms19123785

[58] Djukic T, Simic T, Pljesa-Ercegovac M, Matic M, Suvakov S, Coric V, et al. Upregulated glutathione transferase omega-1 correlates with progression of urinary bladder carcinoma. Redox Report. 2017;**22**:486-492. DOI: 10.1080/13510002.2017.1299909

[59] Govindaraju V, Young K, Maudsley AA. Proton NMR chemical shifts and coupling constants for brain metabolites. NMR in Biomedicine. 2000;**13**:129-153. DOI: 10.1002/1099-1492(200005)13:3<129::aid-nbm619>3.0.co;2-v

[60] Kaiser LG, Marjańska M, Matson GB, Iltis I, Bush SD, Soher BJ, et al. (1)H MRS detection of glycine residue of reduced glutathione in vivo. Journal of Magnetic Resonance. 2010;**202**:259-266. DOI: 10.1016/j.jmr.2009.11.013

[61] Shah N, Sattar A, Benanti M, Hollander S, Cheuck L. Magnetic resonance spectroscopy as an imaging tool for cancer: A review of the literature. The Journal of the American Osteopathic Association. 2006;**106**:23-27

[62] García-Figueiras R, Baleato-González S, Padhani AR, Oleaga L, Vilanova JC, Luna A, et al. Proton magnetic resonance spectroscopy in oncology: The fingerprints of cancer? Diagnostic and Interventional Radiology. 2016;**22**:75-89. DOI: 10.5152/dir.2015.15009